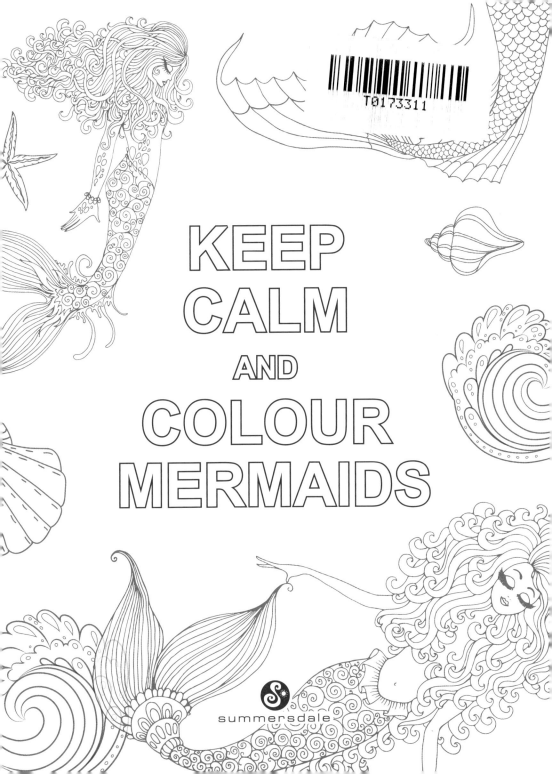

KEEP CALM
AND
COLOUR
MERMAIDS

summersdale

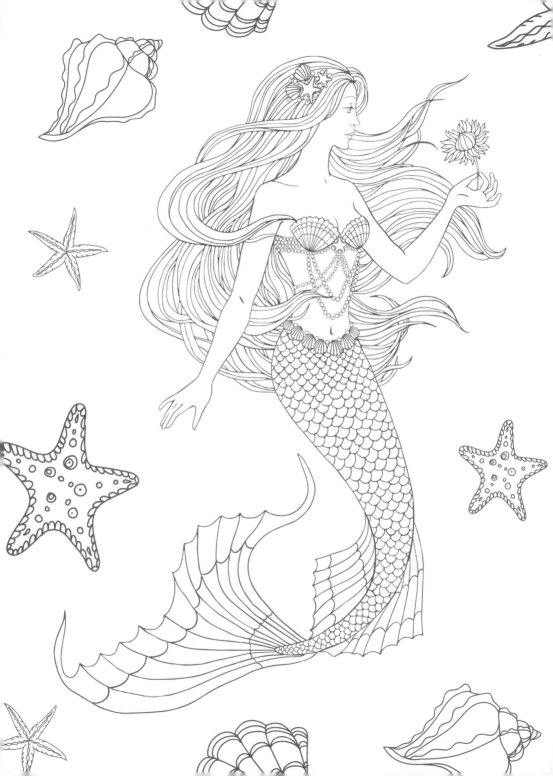

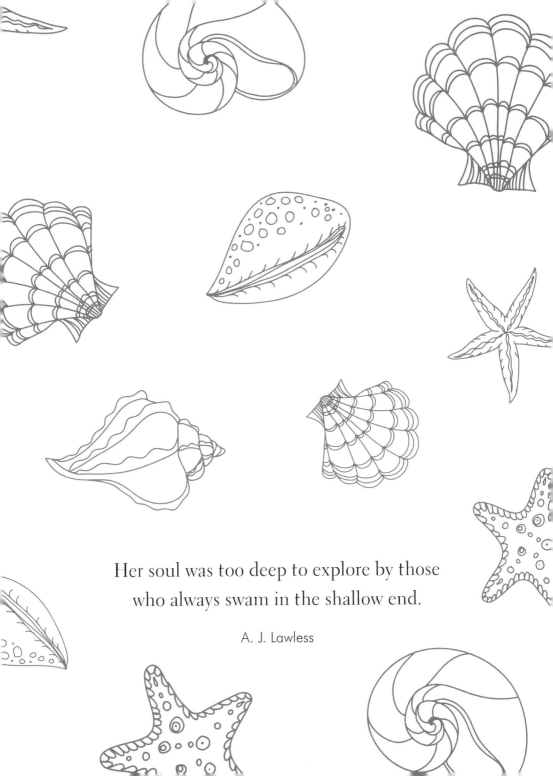

Her soul was too deep to explore by those who always swam in the shallow end.

A. J. Lawless

Land is the secure ground of home, the sea
is like life, the outside, the unknown.

Stephen Gardiner

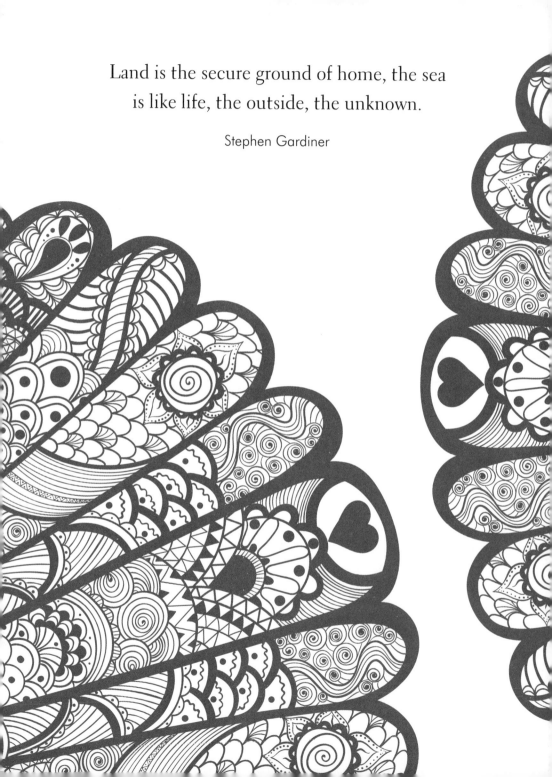

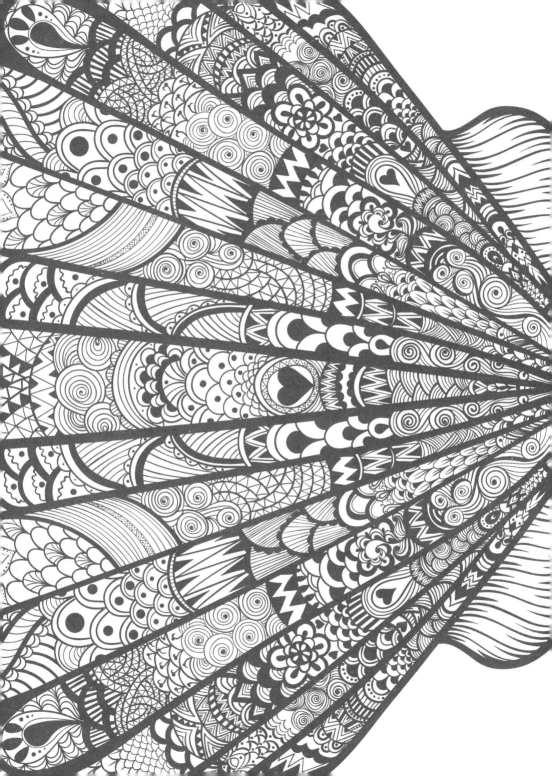

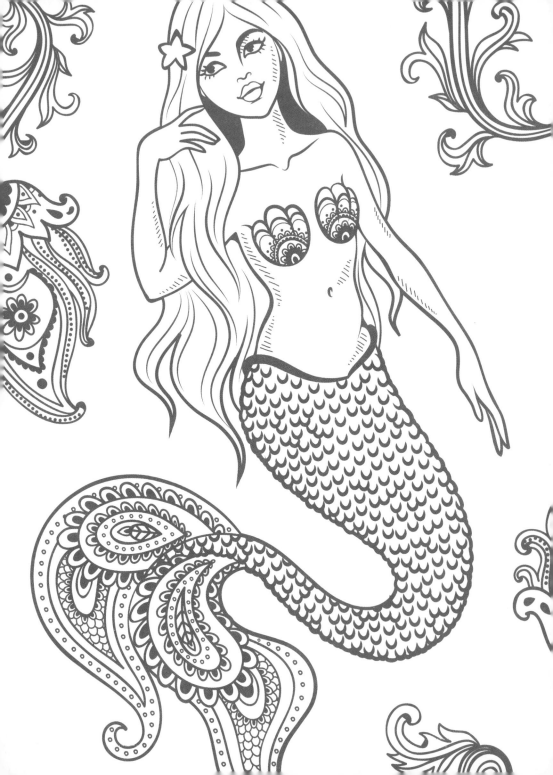

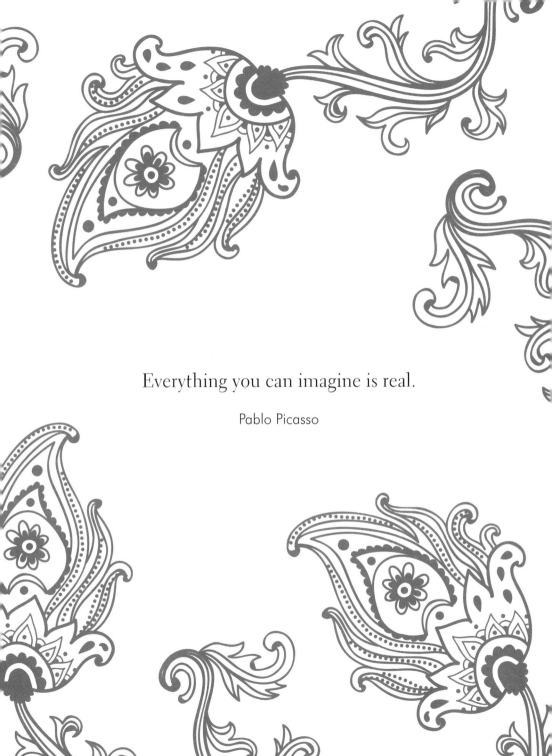

Everything you can imagine is real.

Pablo Picasso

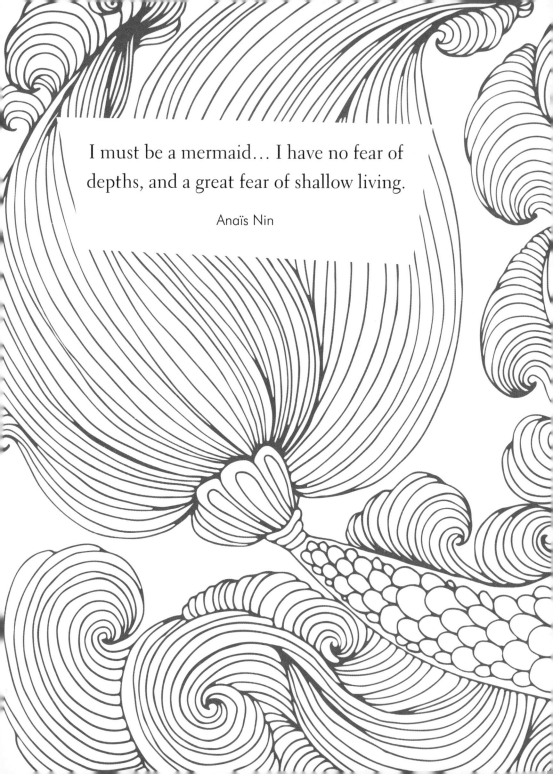

I must be a mermaid… I have no fear of depths, and a great fear of shallow living.

Anaïs Nin

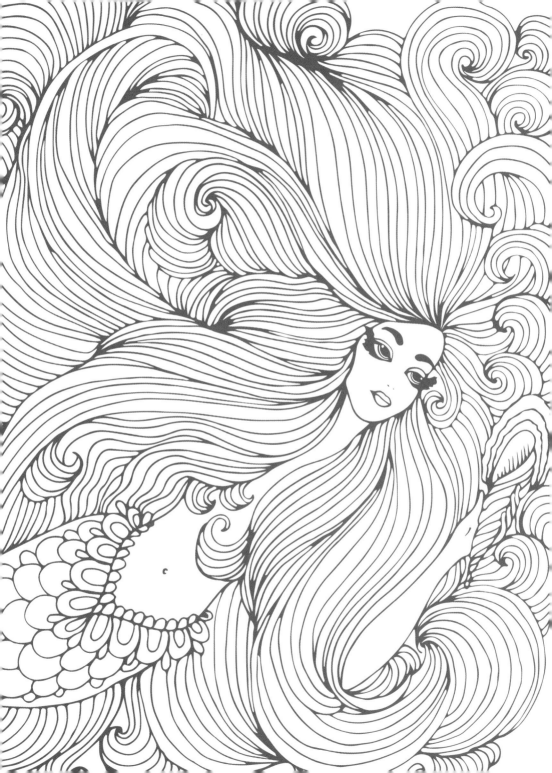

The sea, once it casts its spell, holds
one in its net of wonder forever.

Jacques Cousteau

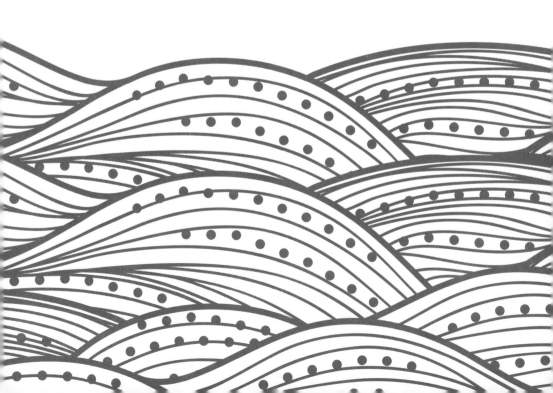

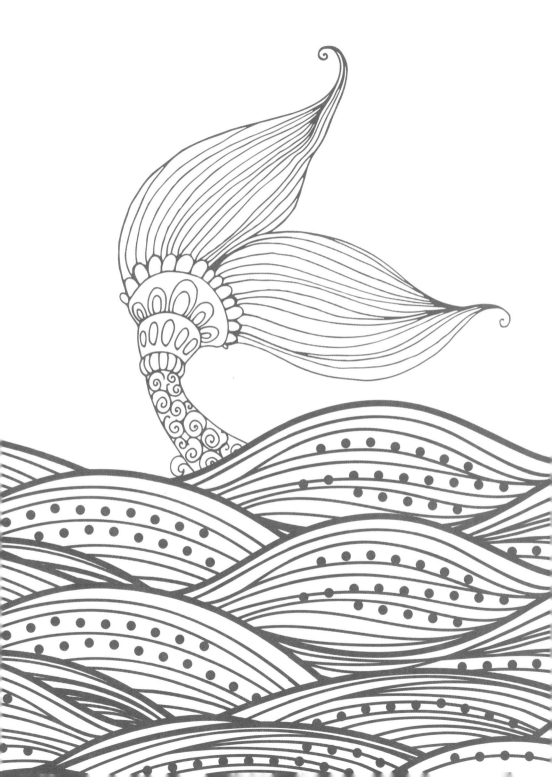

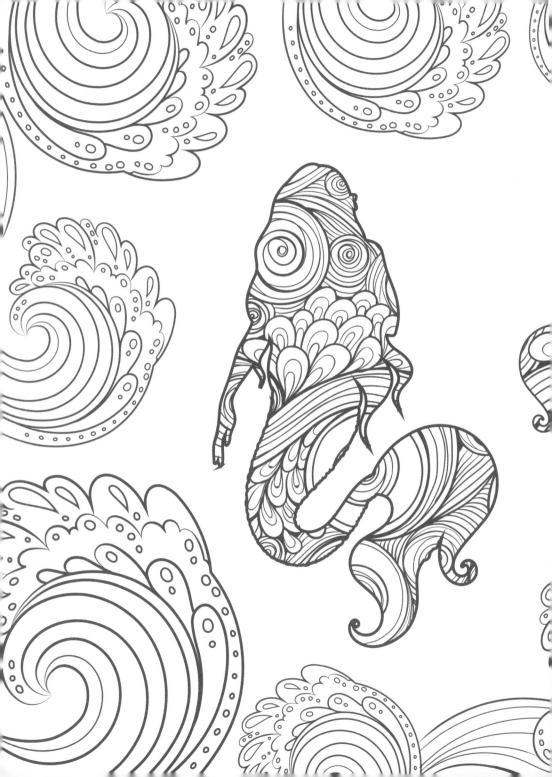

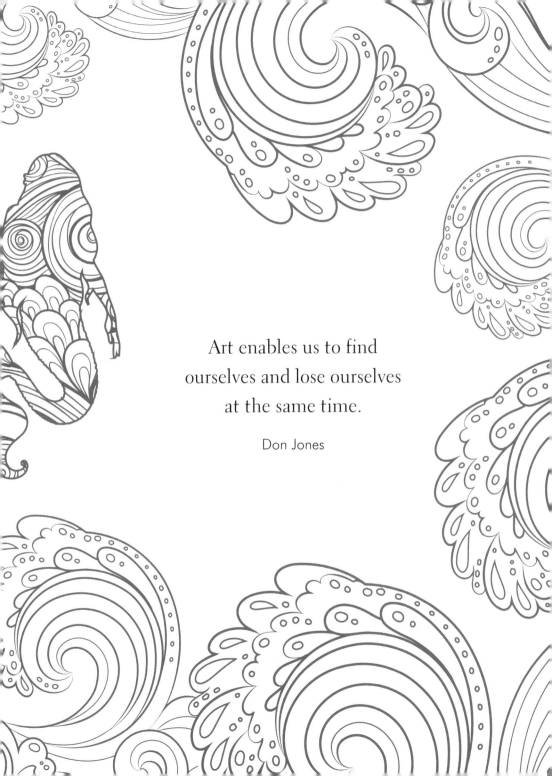

Art enables us to find
ourselves and lose ourselves
at the same time.

Don Jones

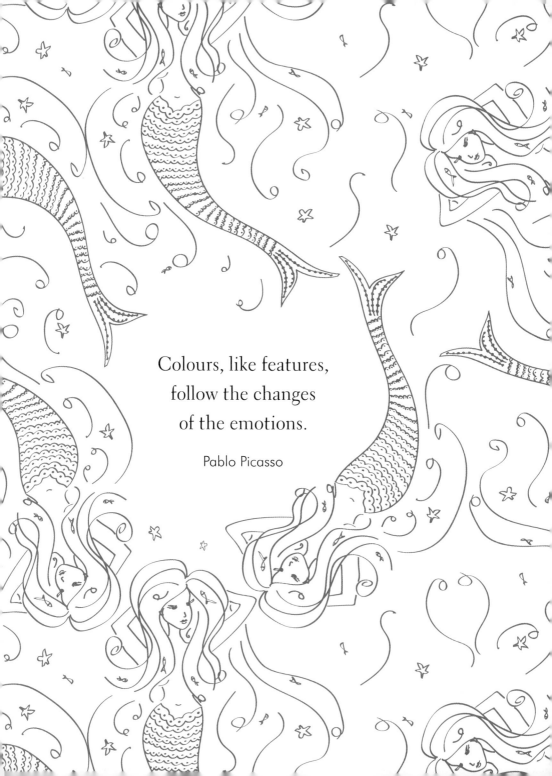

Colours, like features,
follow the changes
of the emotions.

Pablo Picasso

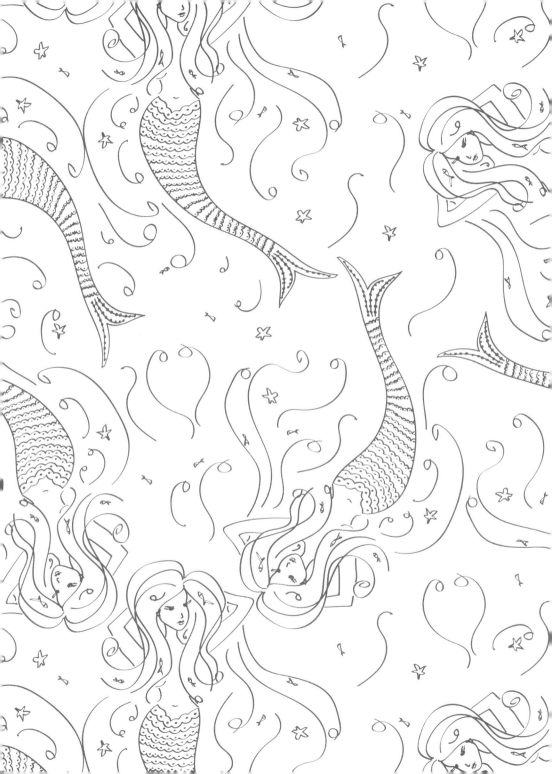

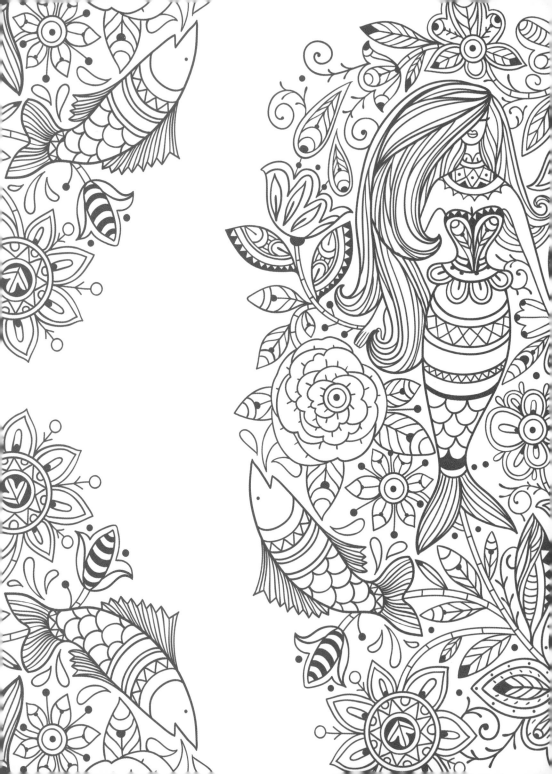

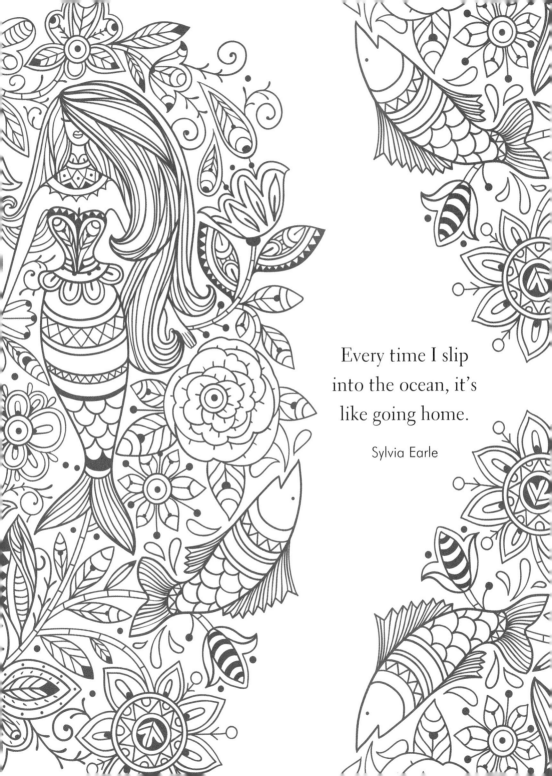

Every time I slip
into the ocean, it's
like going home.

Sylvia Earle

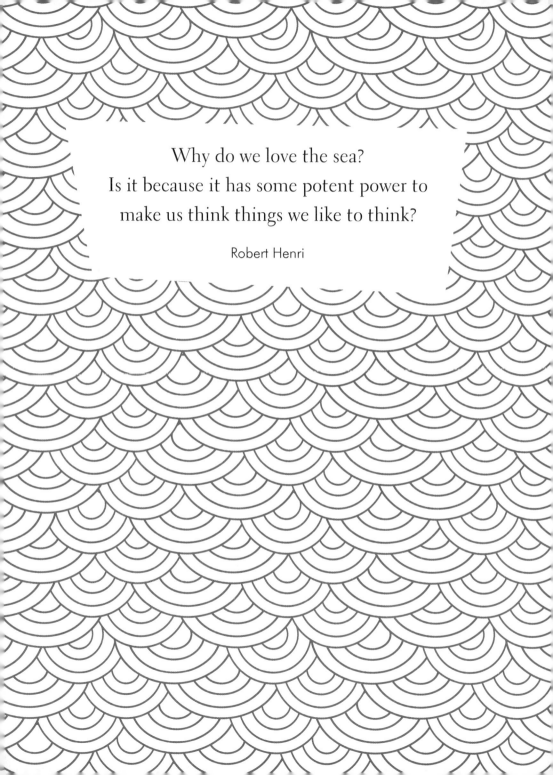

Why do we love the sea?
Is it because it has some potent power to
make us think things we like to think?

Robert Henri

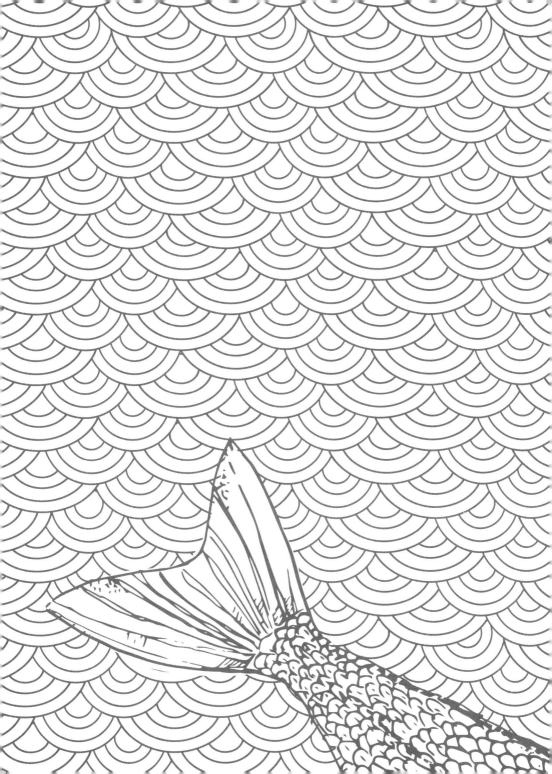

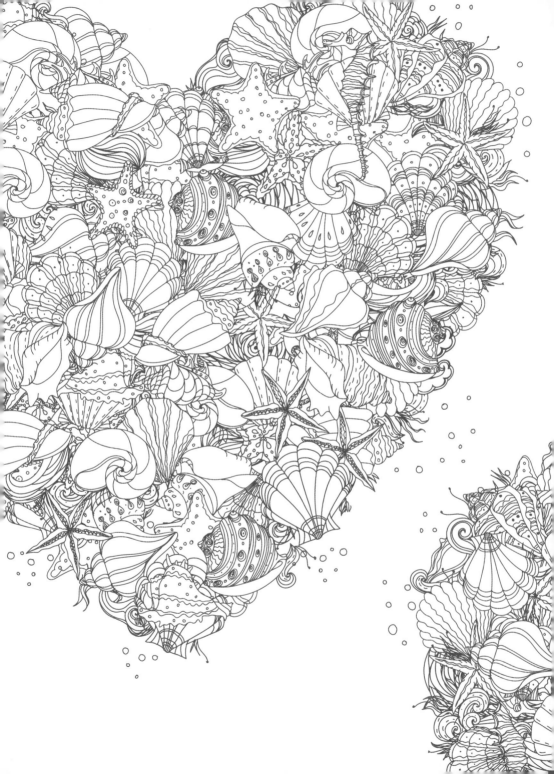

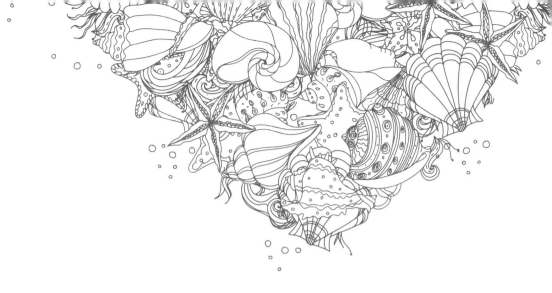

Teach me to hear mermaids singing.

John Donne

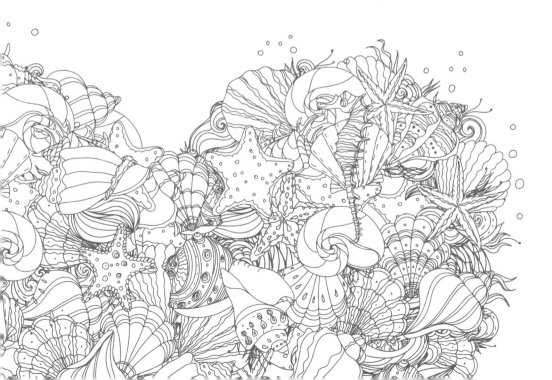

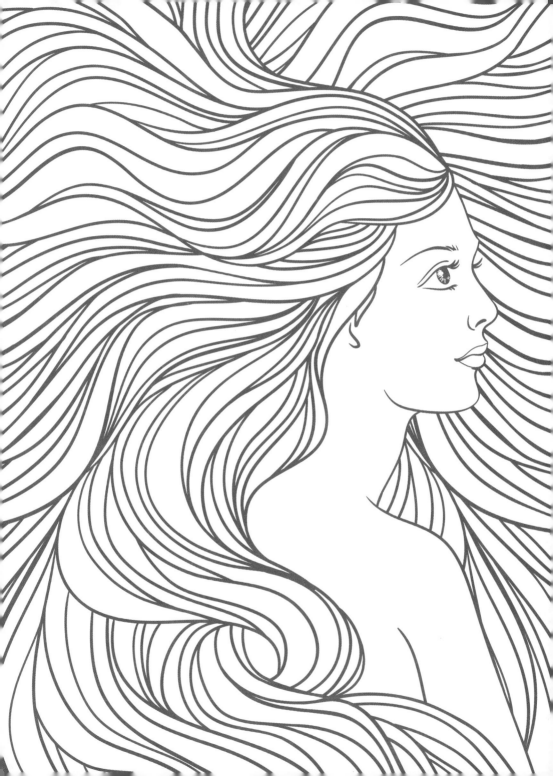

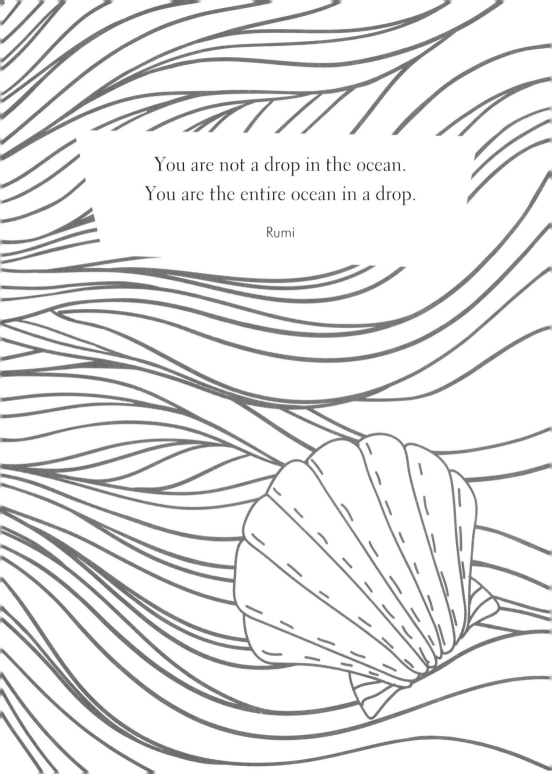

You are not a drop in the ocean.
You are the entire ocean in a drop.

Rumi

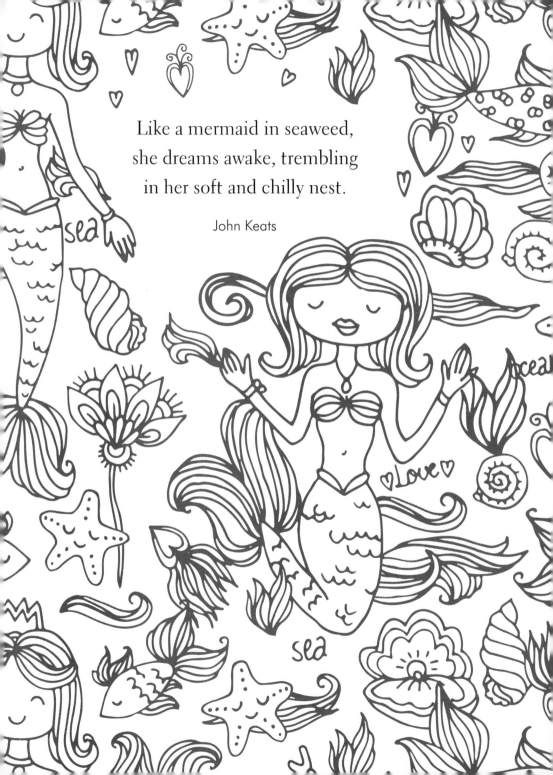

Like a mermaid in seaweed,
she dreams awake, trembling
in her soft and chilly nest.

John Keats

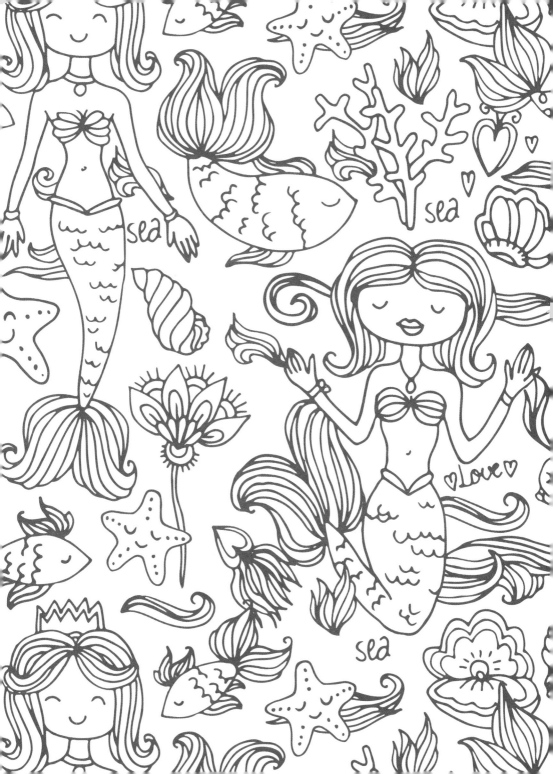

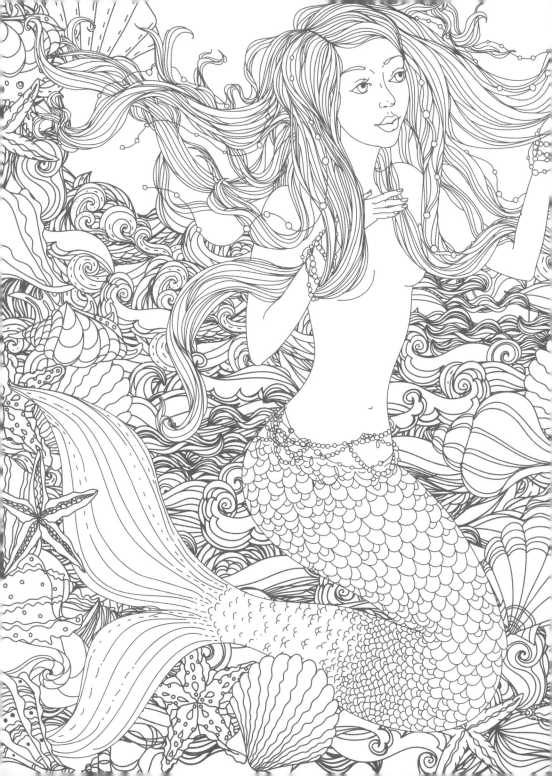

Daydreaming with
pencil and paper is
a respectable form
of meditation.

John Howe

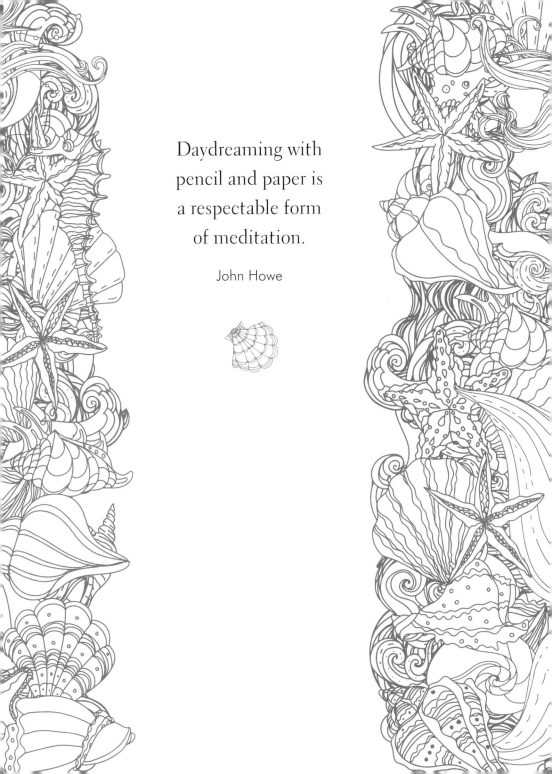

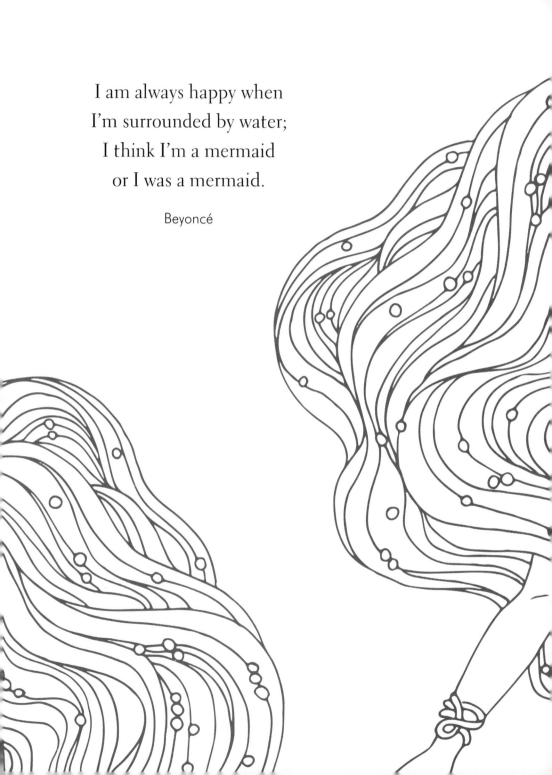

I am always happy when
I'm surrounded by water;
I think I'm a mermaid
or I was a mermaid.

Beyoncé

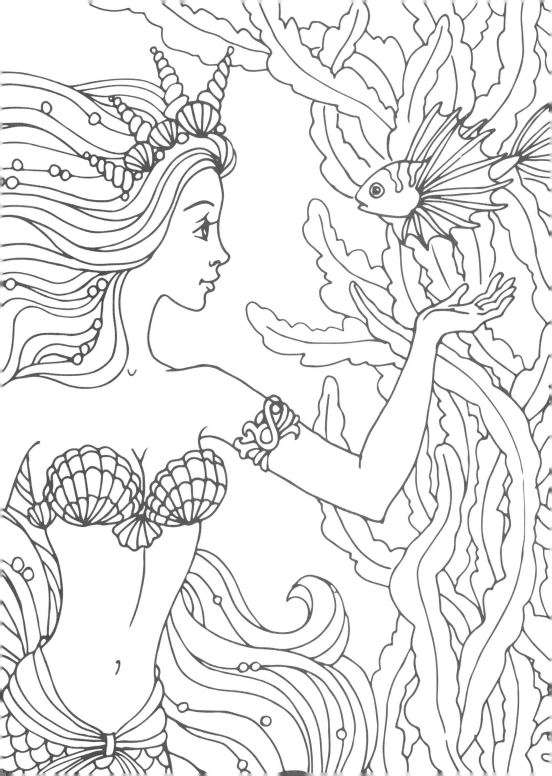

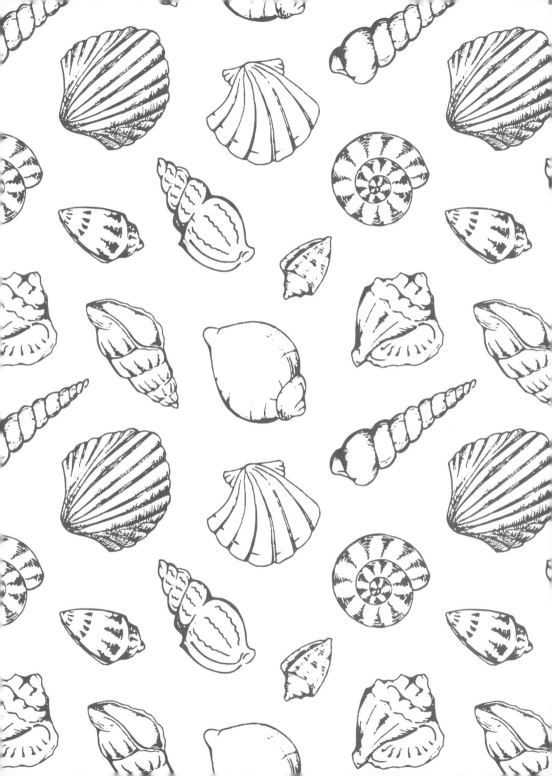

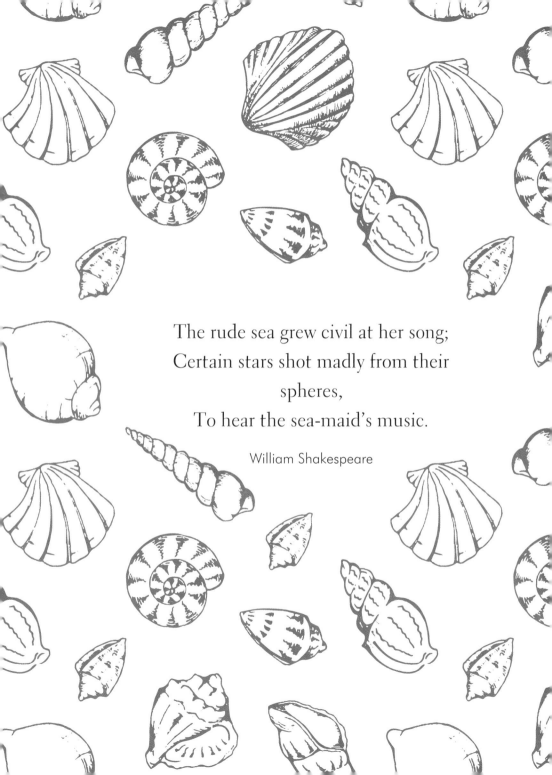

The rude sea grew civil at her song;
Certain stars shot madly from their
spheres,
To hear the sea-maid's music.

William Shakespeare

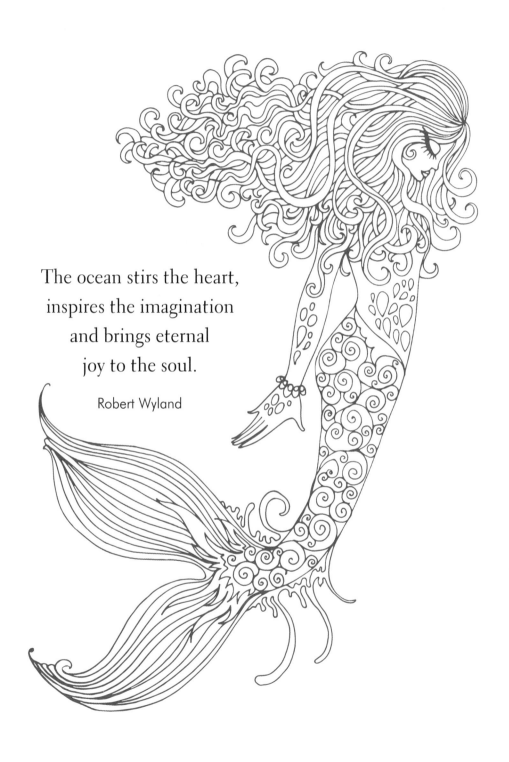

The ocean stirs the heart,
inspires the imagination
and brings eternal
joy to the soul.

Robert Wyland

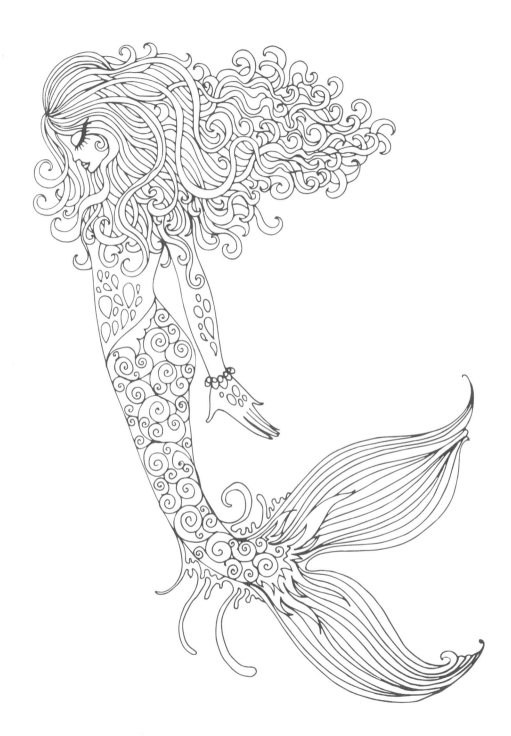

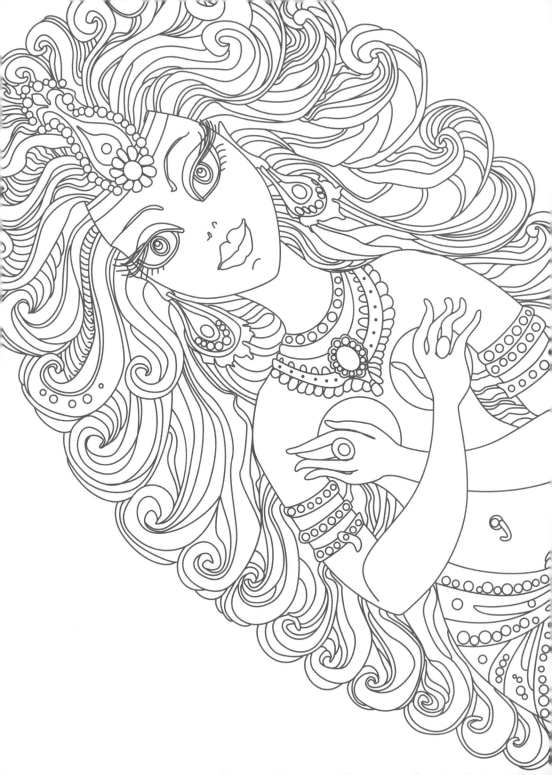

The sea hath no
king but God alone.

Dante Gabriel Rossetti

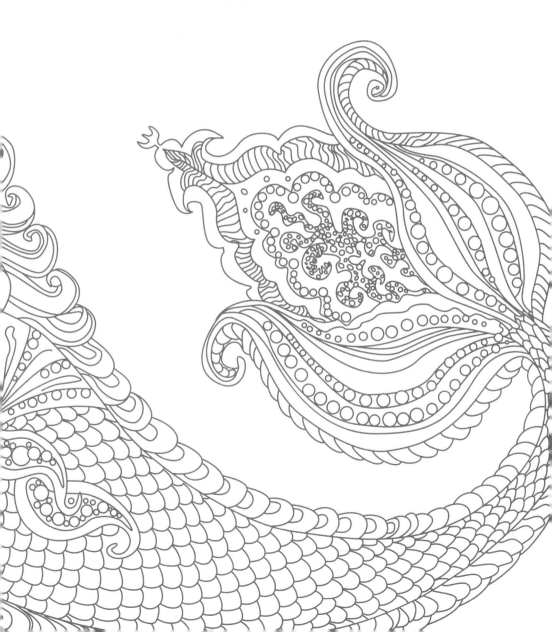

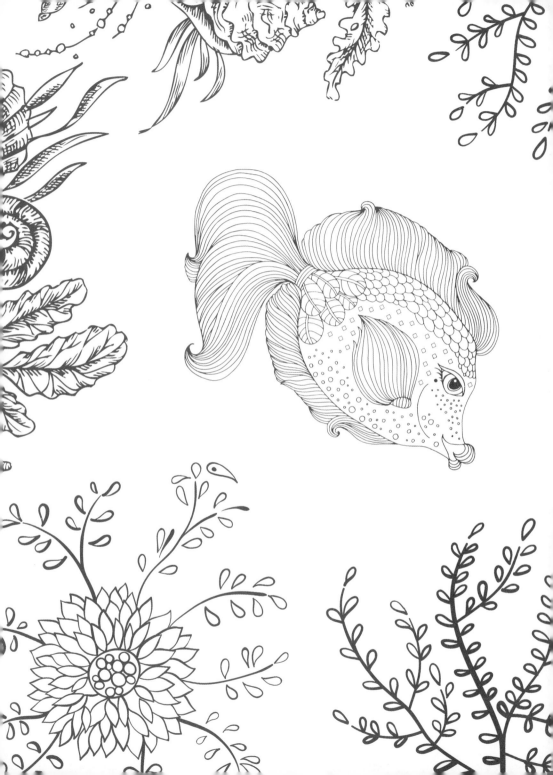

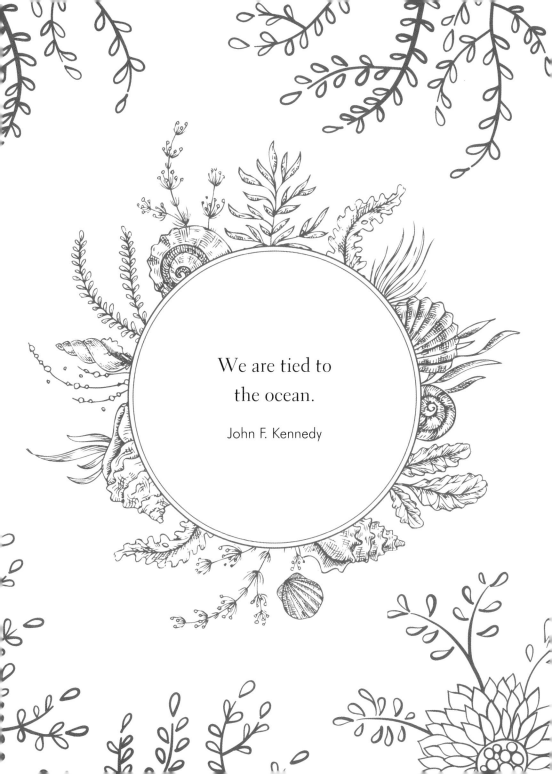

We are tied to
the ocean.

John F. Kennedy

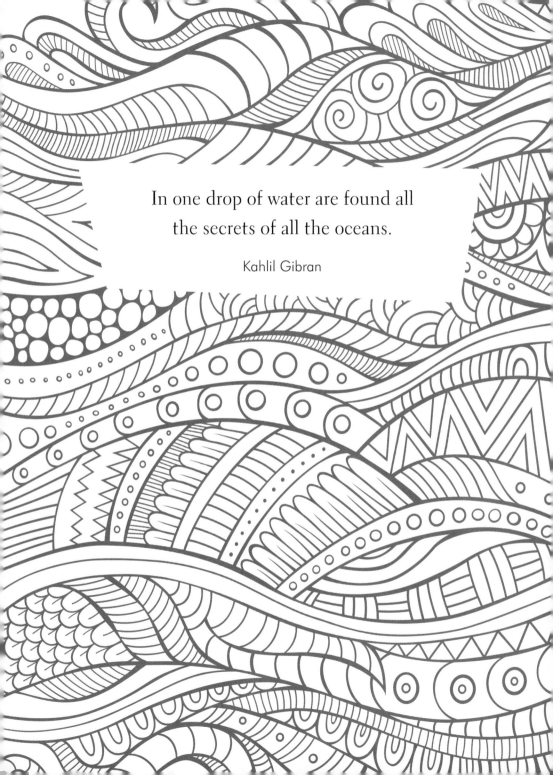

In one drop of water are found all
the secrets of all the oceans.

Kahlil Gibran

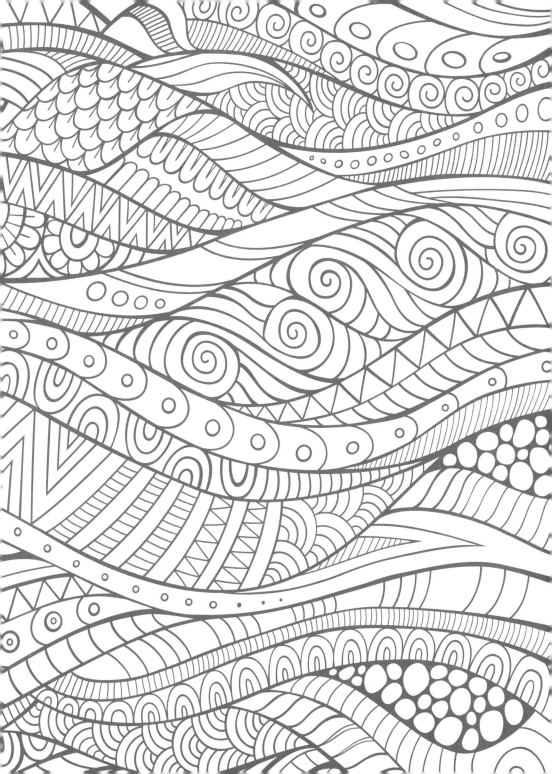

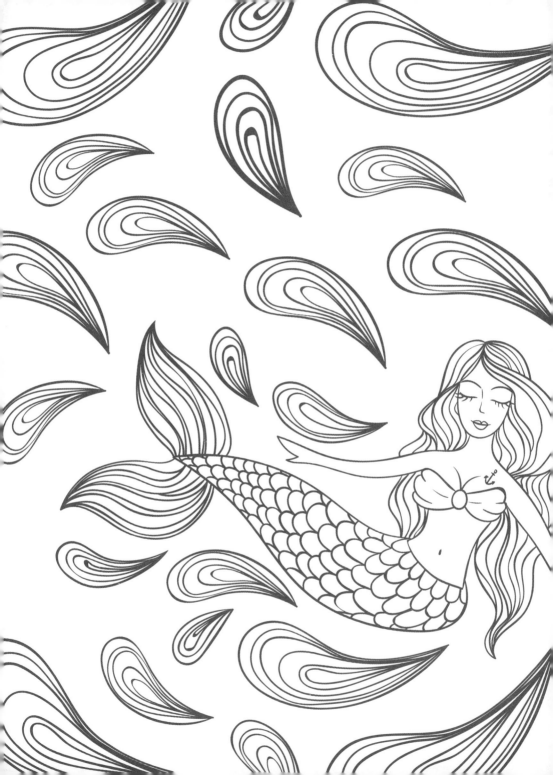

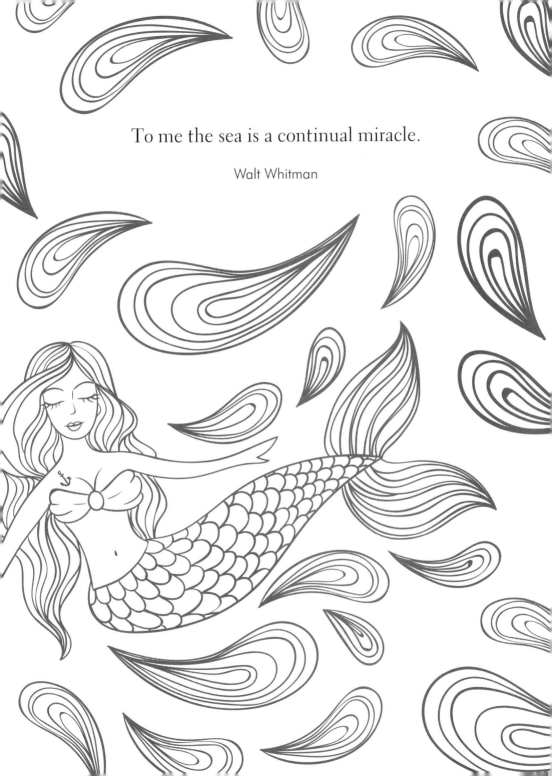

To me the sea is a continual miracle.

Walt Whitman

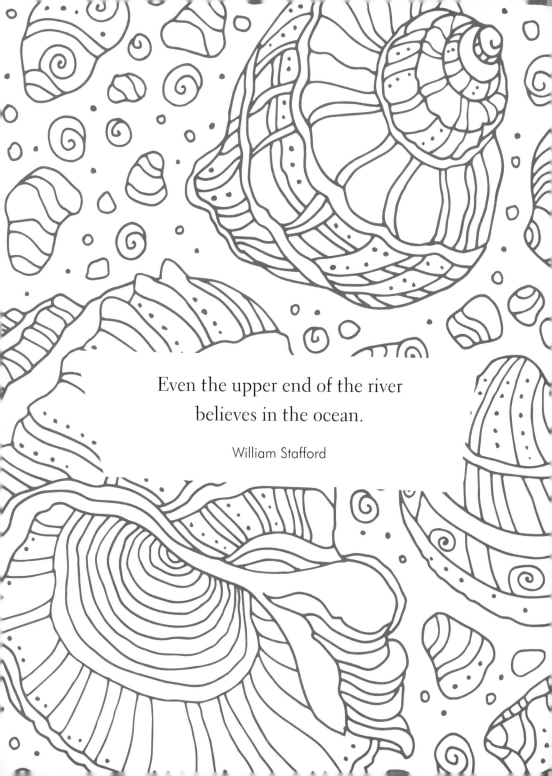

Even the upper end of the river
believes in the ocean.

William Stafford

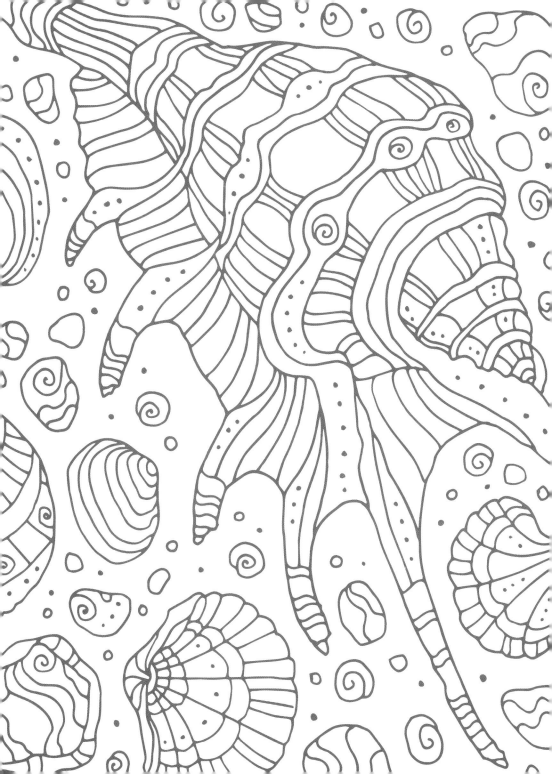

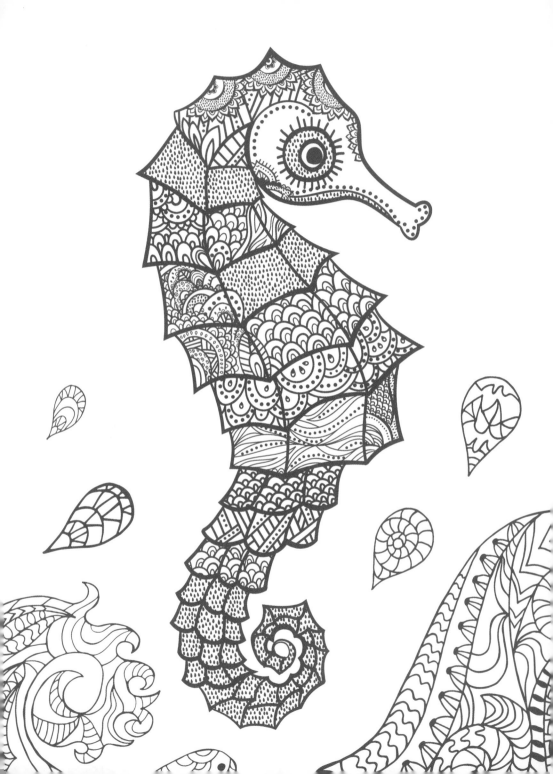

The voice of the sea speaks to the soul.

Kate Chopin

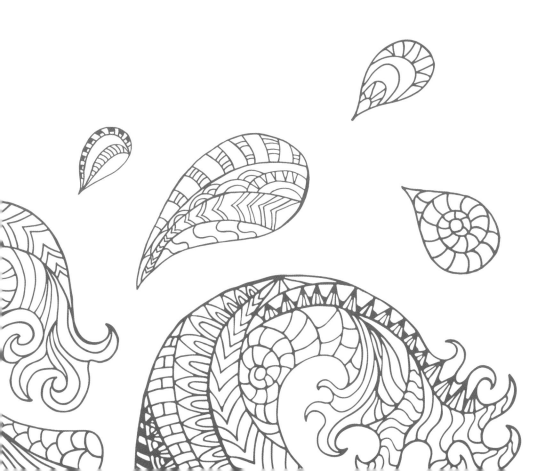

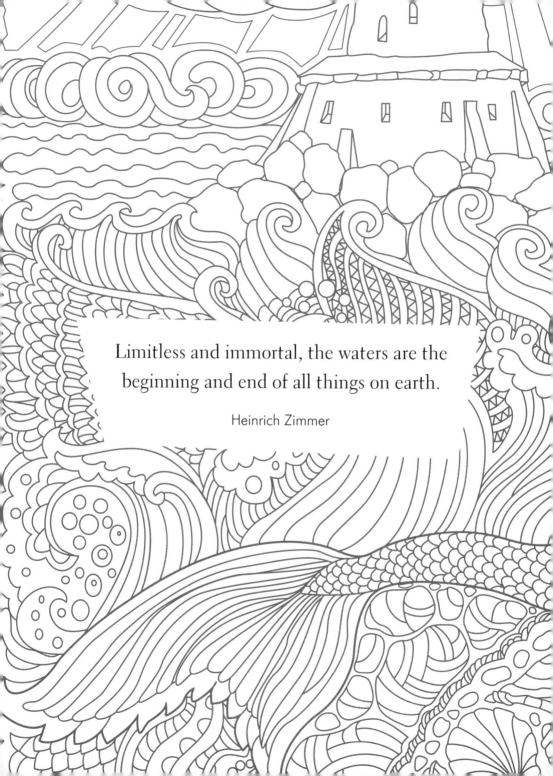

Limitless and immortal, the waters are the beginning and end of all things on earth.

Heinrich Zimmer

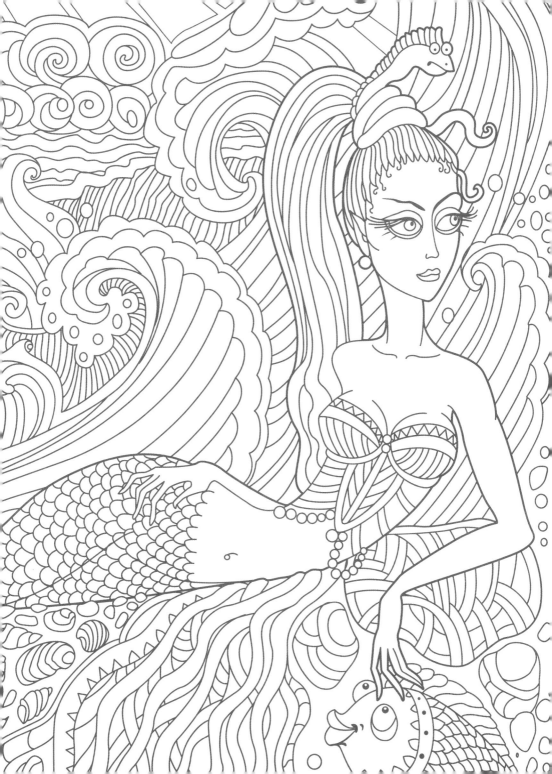

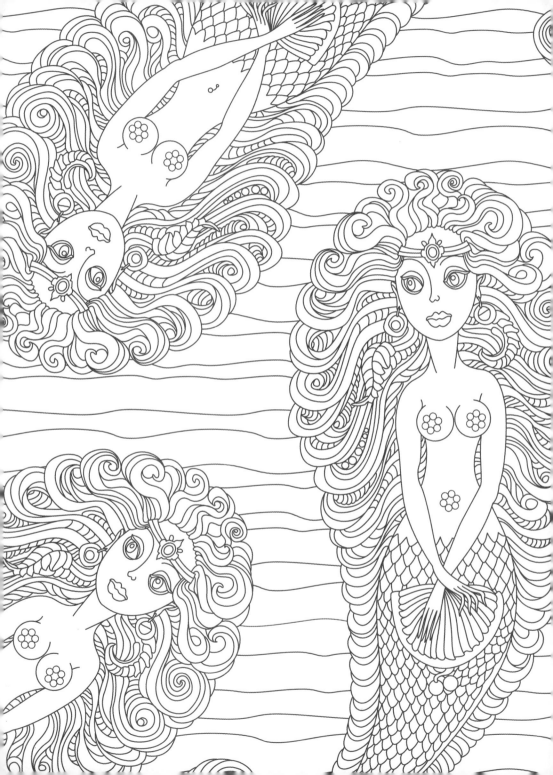

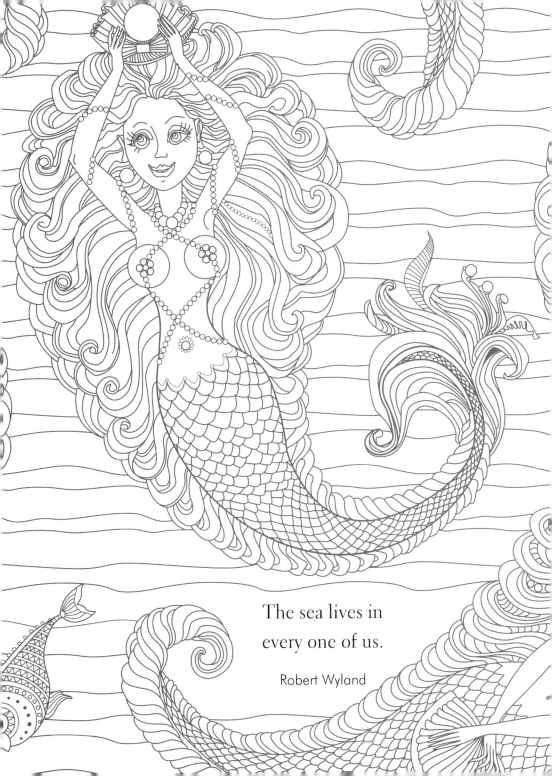

The sea lives in
every one of us.

Robert Wyland

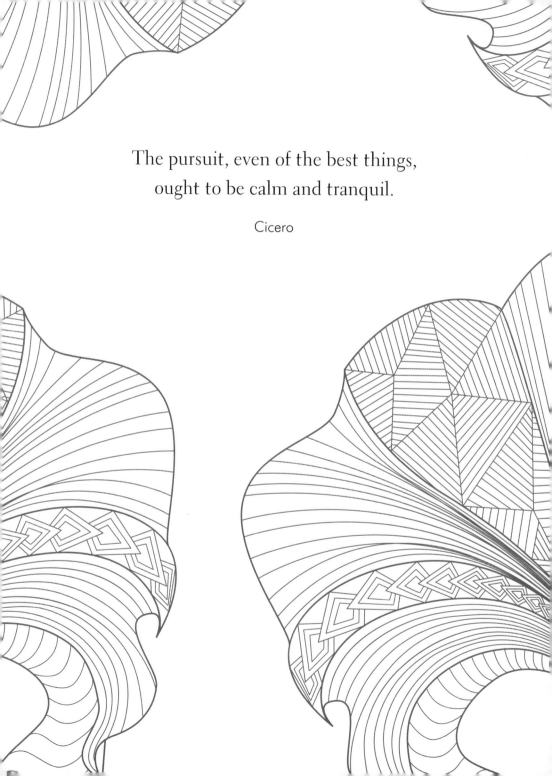

The pursuit, even of the best things,
ought to be calm and tranquil.

Cicero

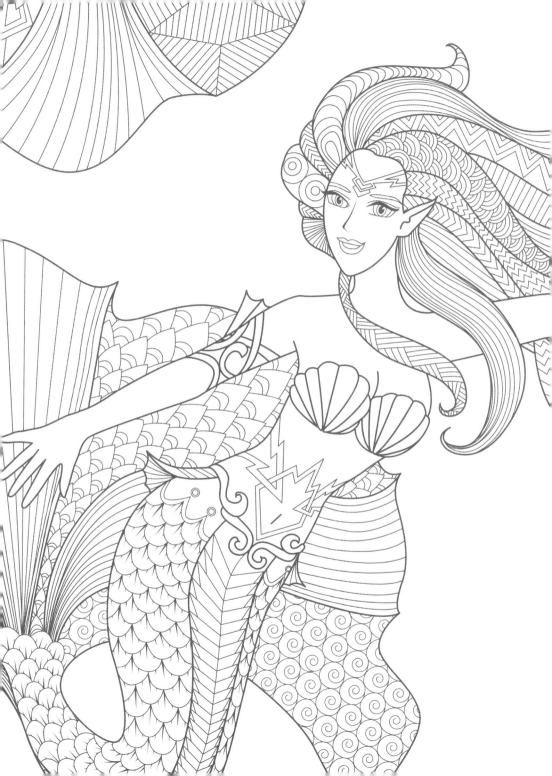

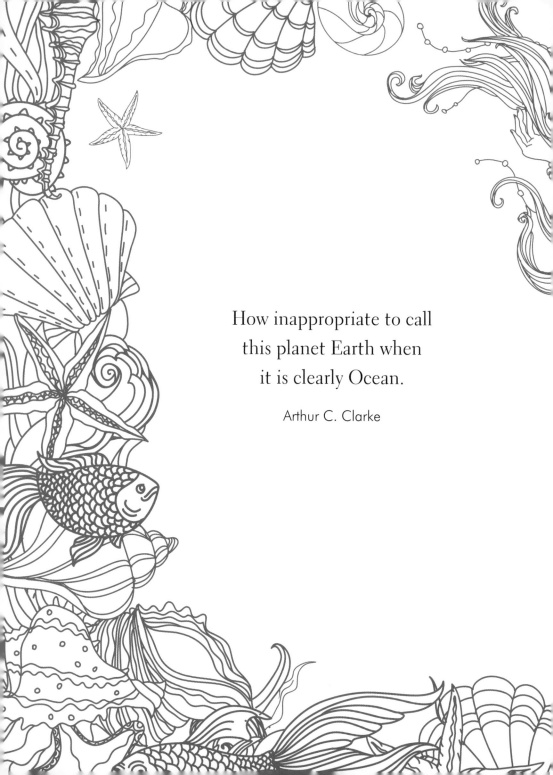

How inappropriate to call
this planet Earth when
it is clearly Ocean.

Arthur C. Clarke

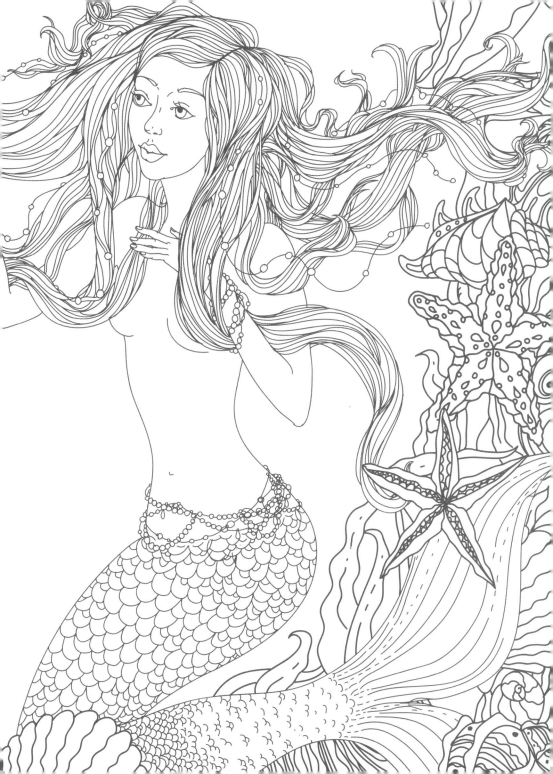

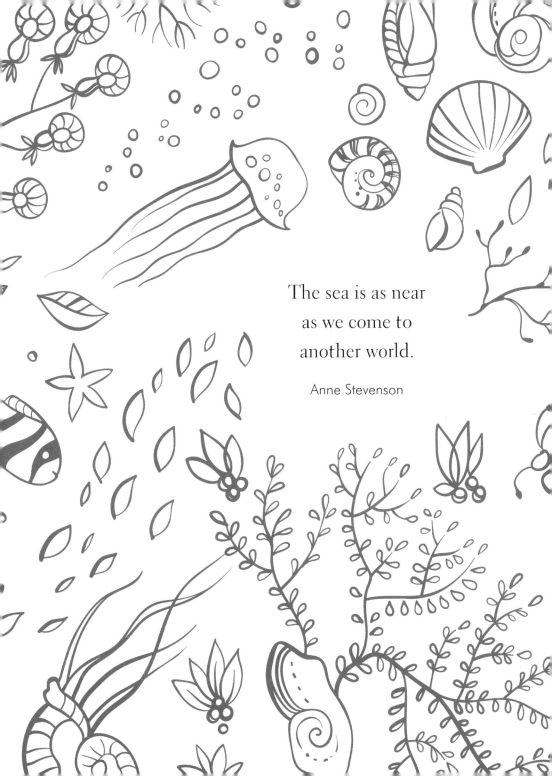

The sea is as near
as we come to
another world.

Anne Stevenson

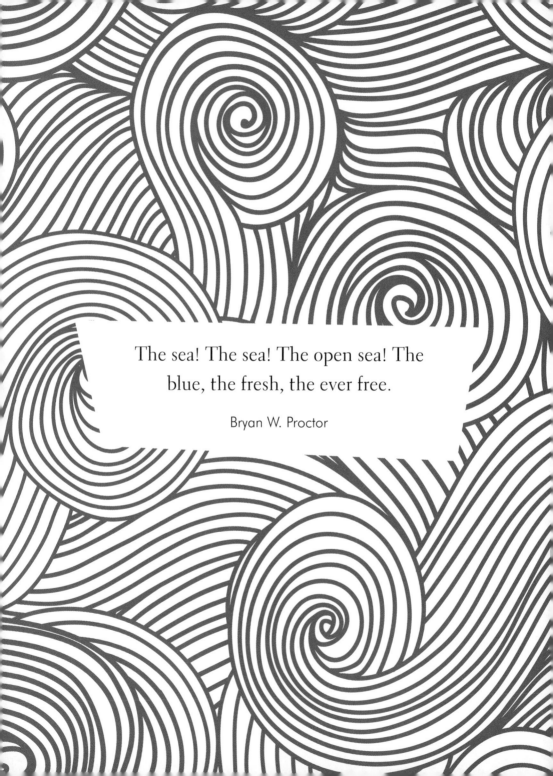

The sea! The sea! The open sea! The blue, the fresh, the ever free.

Bryan W. Proctor

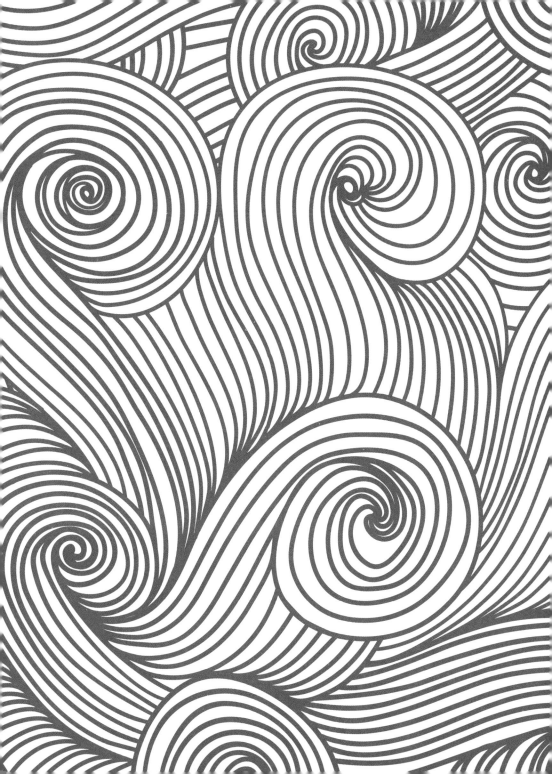

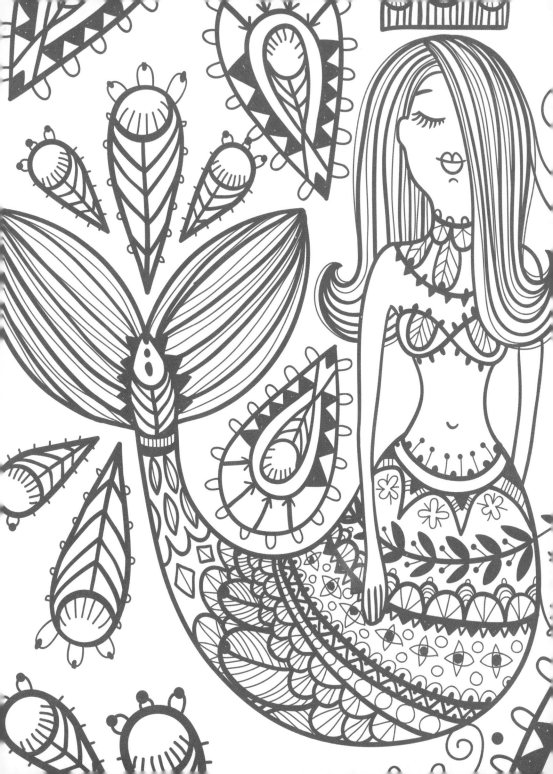

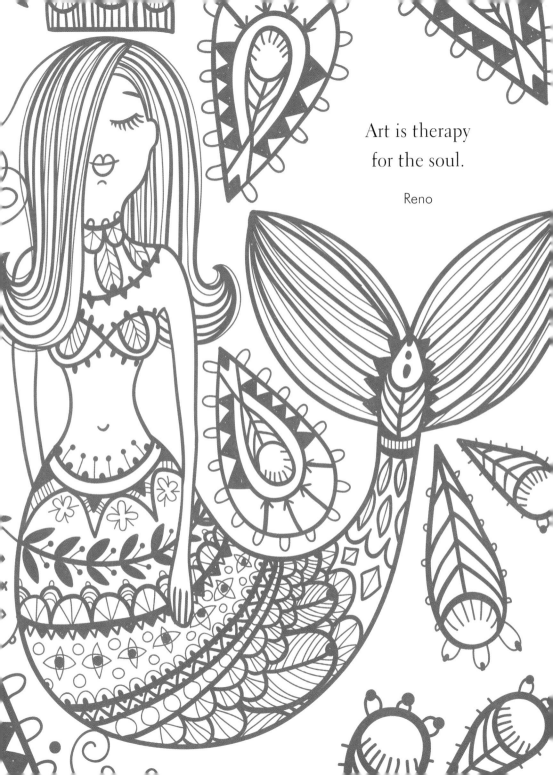

Art is therapy
for the soul.

Reno

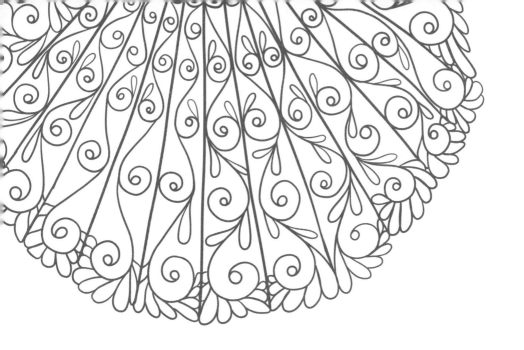

Make your story so beautiful mermaids
have trouble believing it's true.

Anonymous

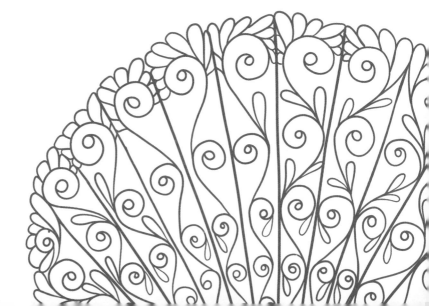

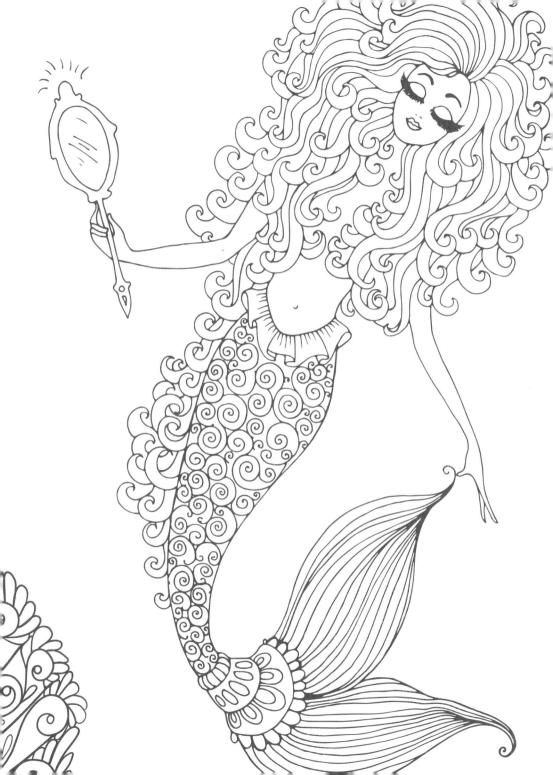

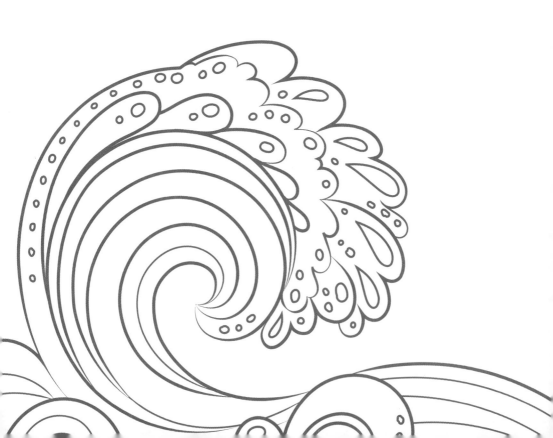

Imagination is everything.
It is the preview of life's
coming attractions.

Albert Einstein

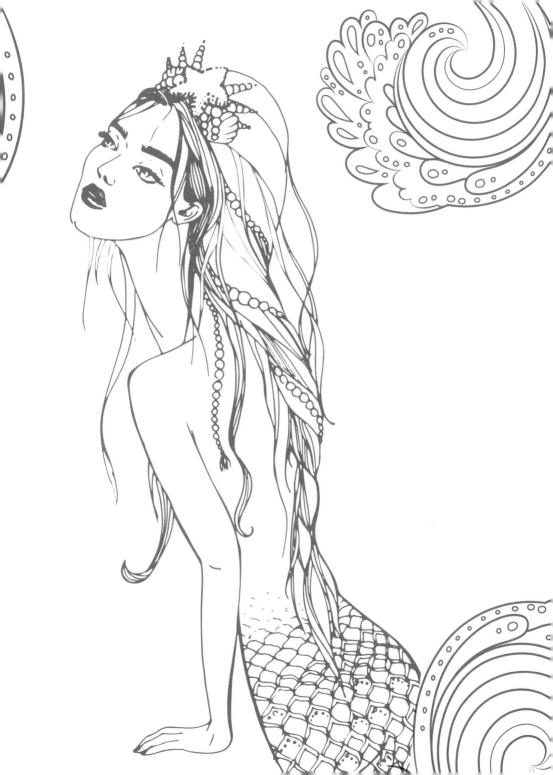

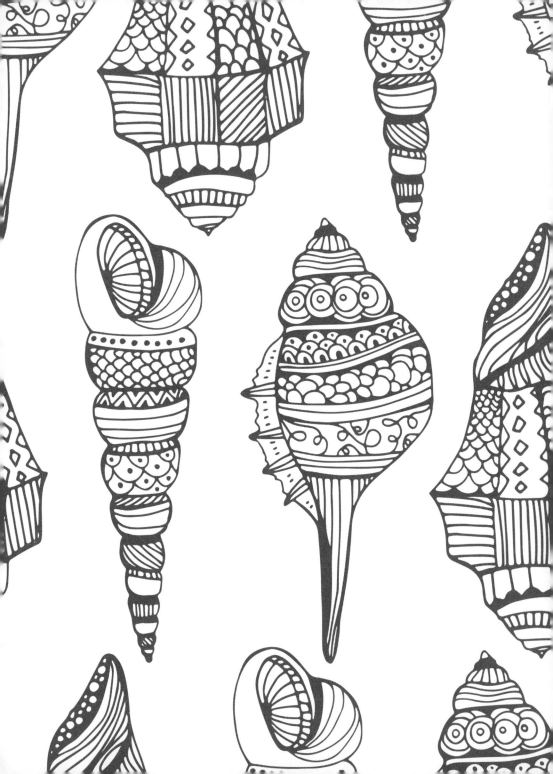

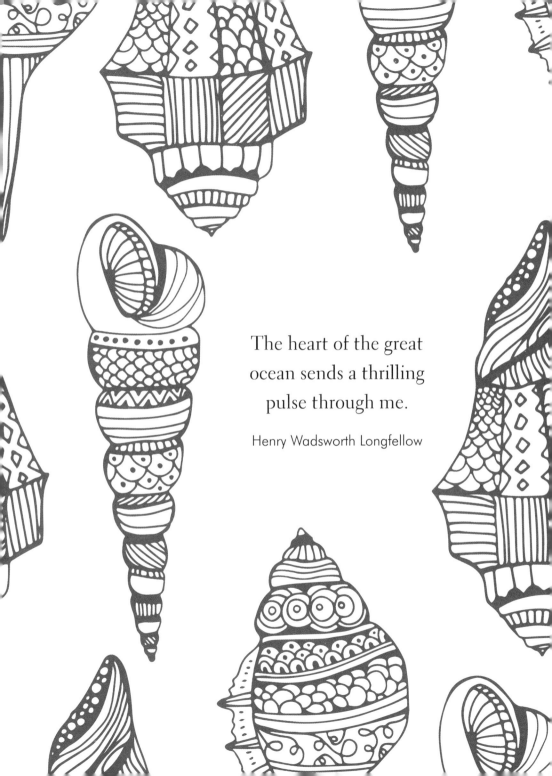

The heart of the great
ocean sends a thrilling
pulse through me.

Henry Wadsworth Longfellow

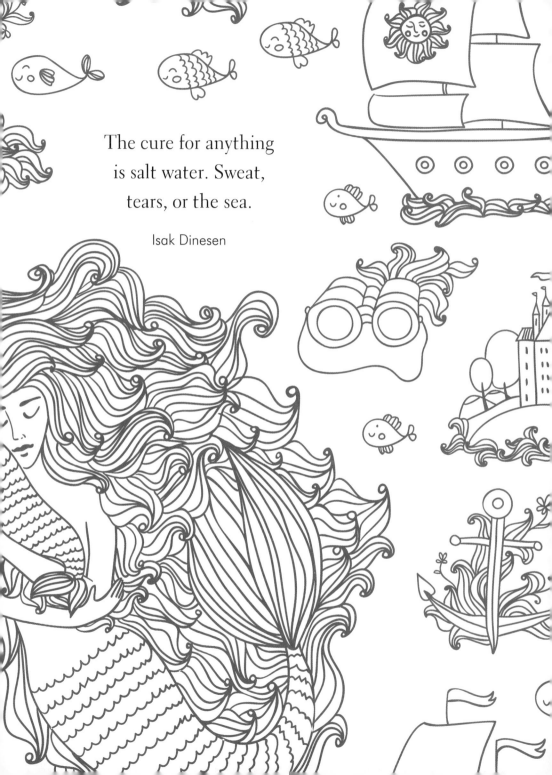

The cure for anything
is salt water. Sweat,
tears, or the sea.

Isak Dinesen

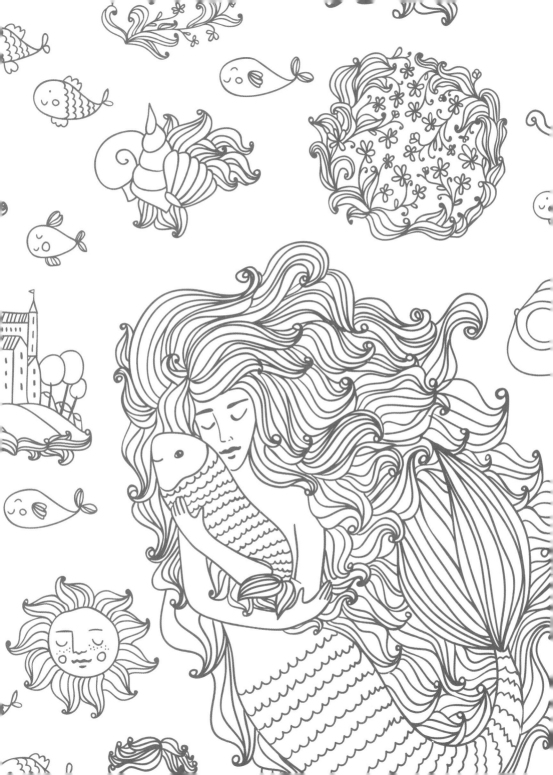

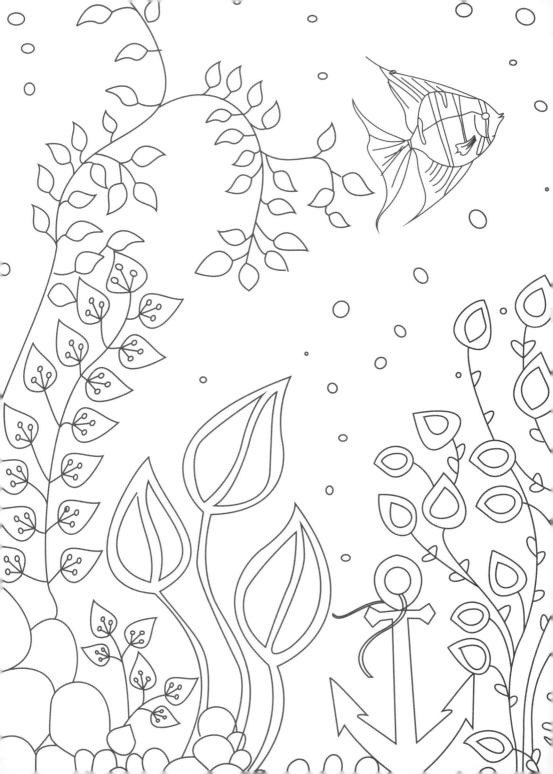

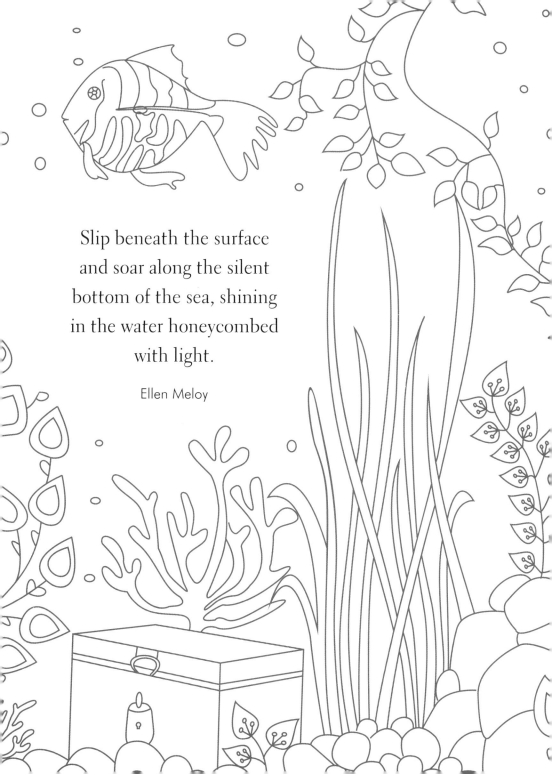

Slip beneath the surface
and soar along the silent
bottom of the sea, shining
in the water honeycombed
with light.

Ellen Meloy

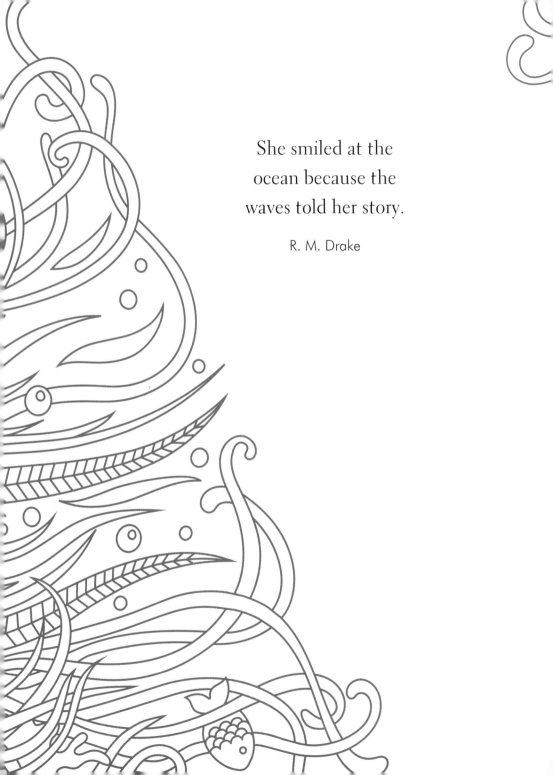

She smiled at the
ocean because the
waves told her story.

R. M. Drake

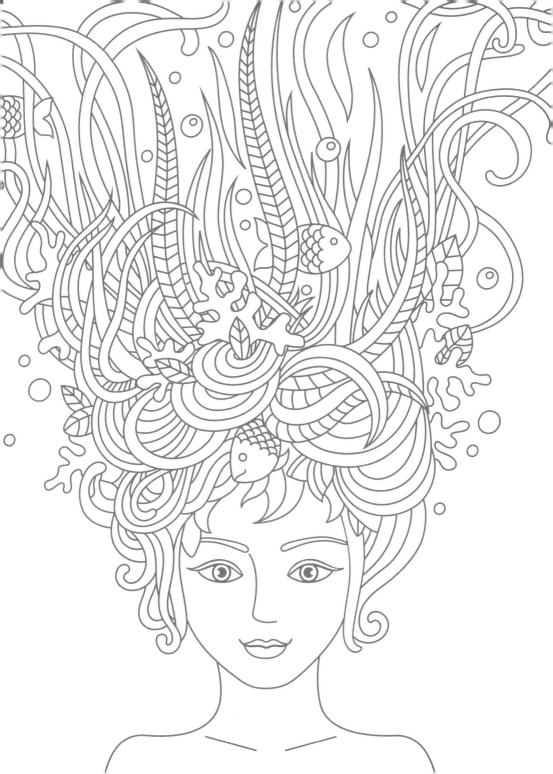

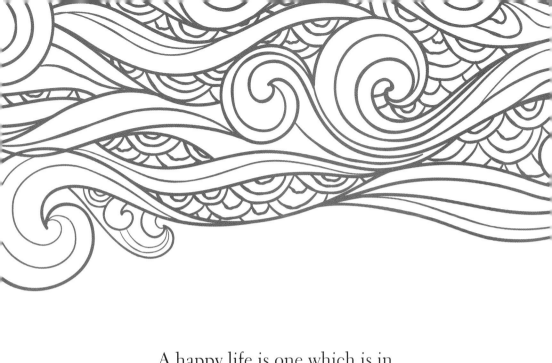

A happy life is one which is in
accordance with its own nature.

Seneca

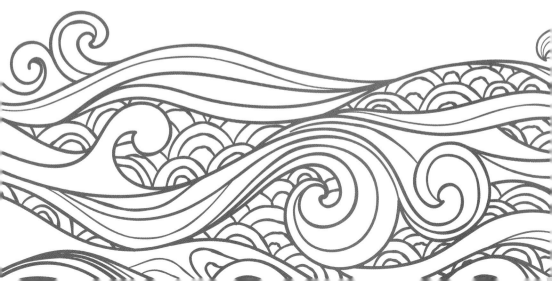

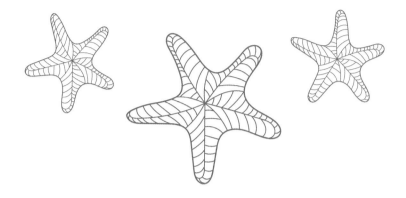

Limitless and immortal,
the waters are the beginning
and end of all things on earth.

Heinrich Zimmer

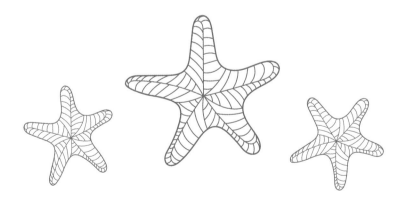

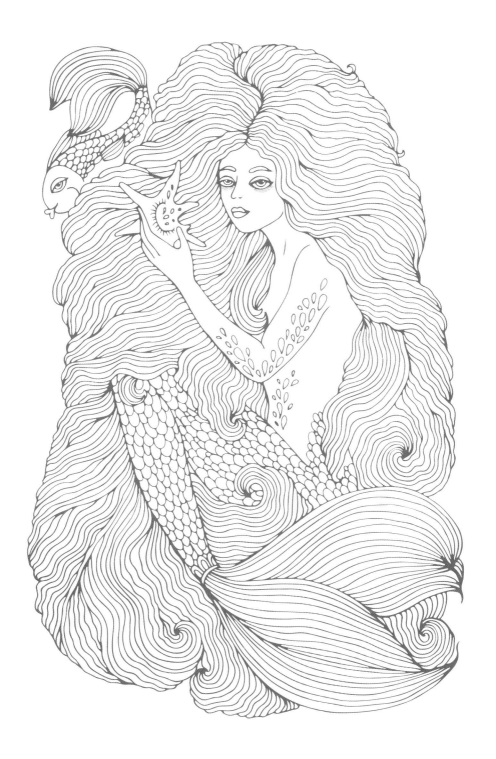

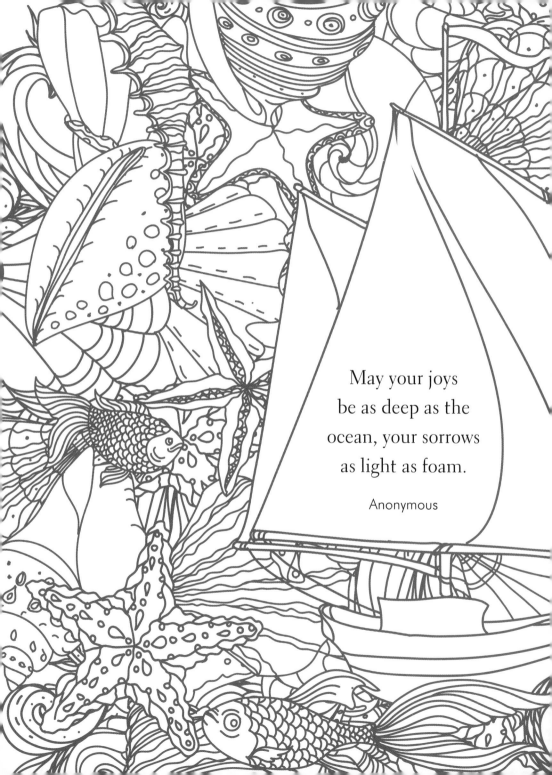

May your joys
be as deep as the
ocean, your sorrows
as light as foam.

Anonymous

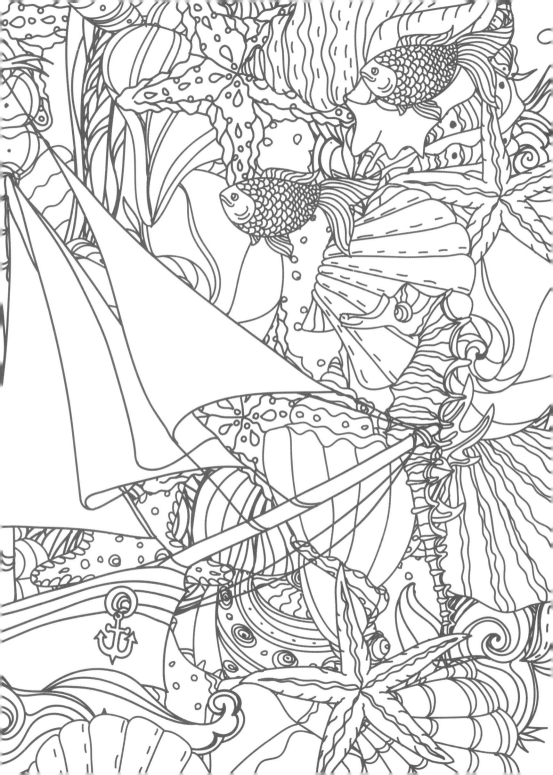

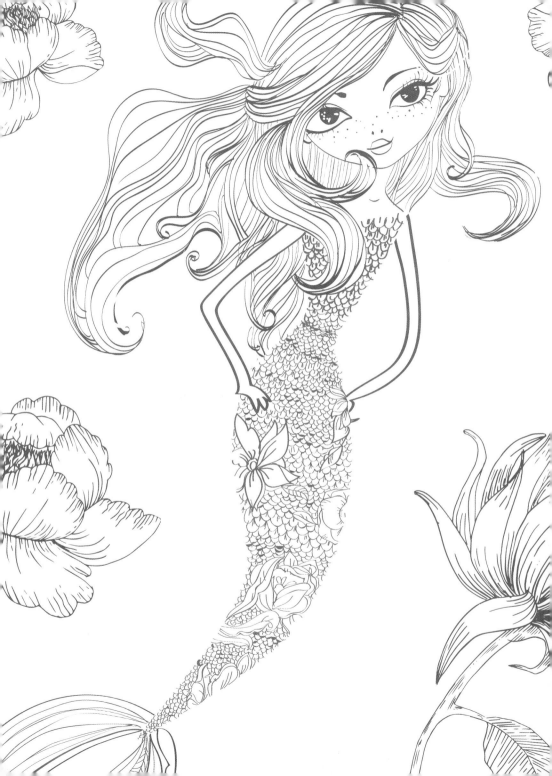

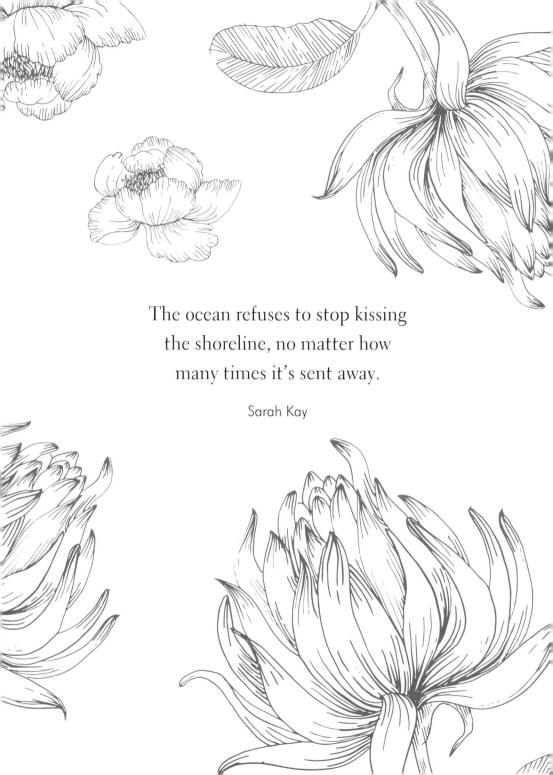

The ocean refuses to stop kissing
the shoreline, no matter how
many times it's sent away.

Sarah Kay

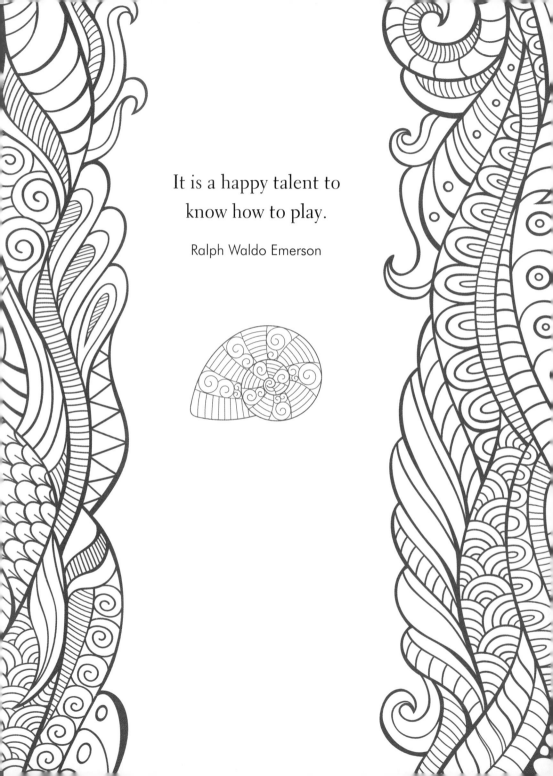

It is a happy talent to
know how to play.

Ralph Waldo Emerson

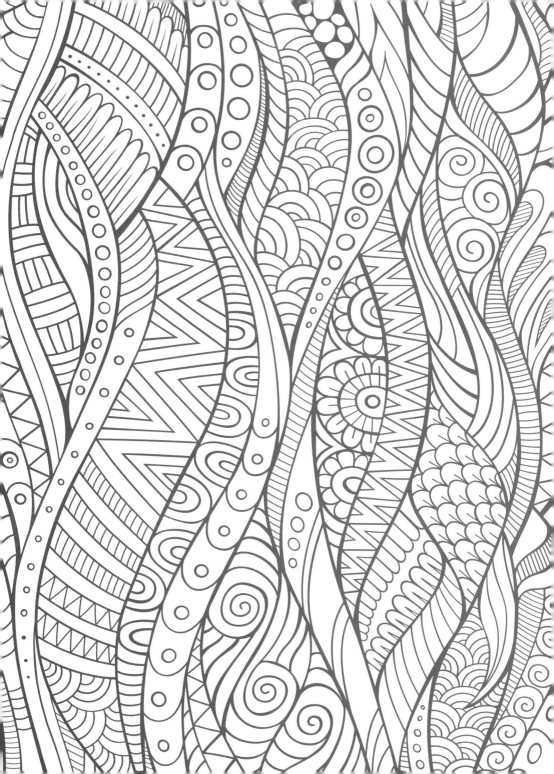

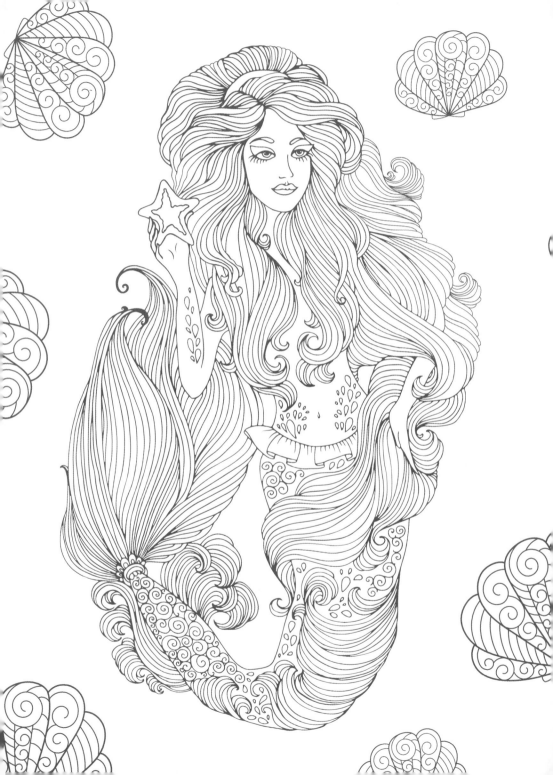

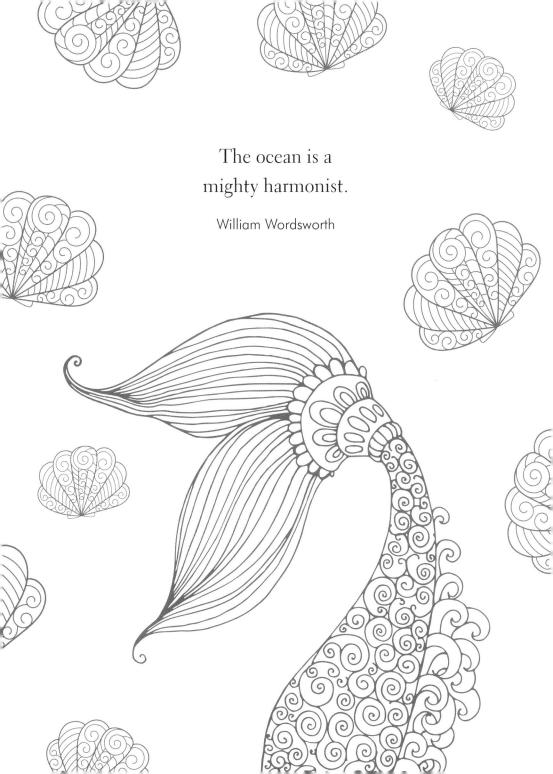

The ocean is a
mighty harmonist.

William Wordsworth

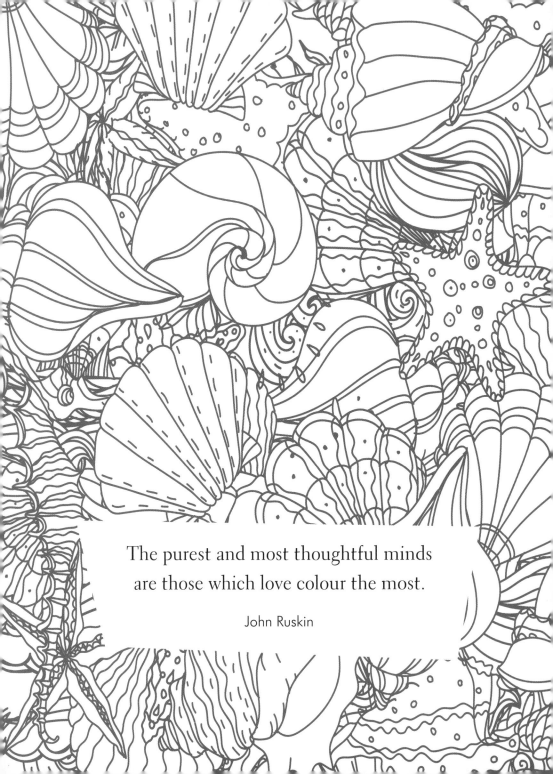

The purest and most thoughtful minds
are those which love colour the most.

John Ruskin

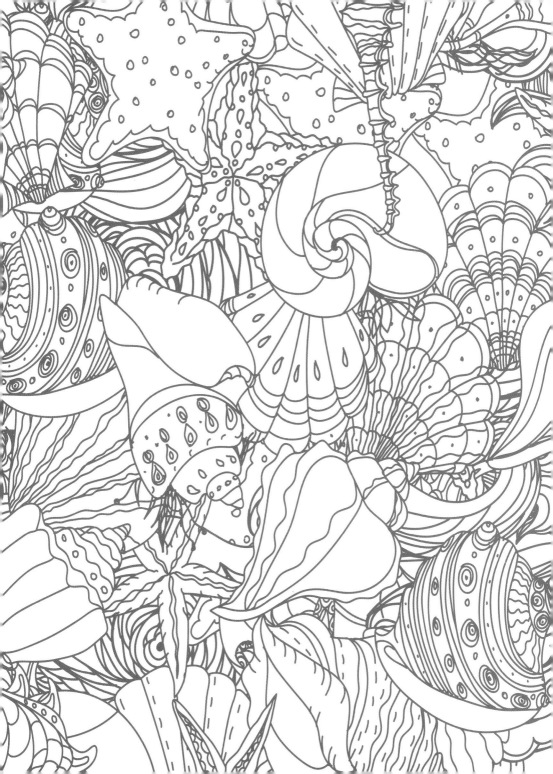

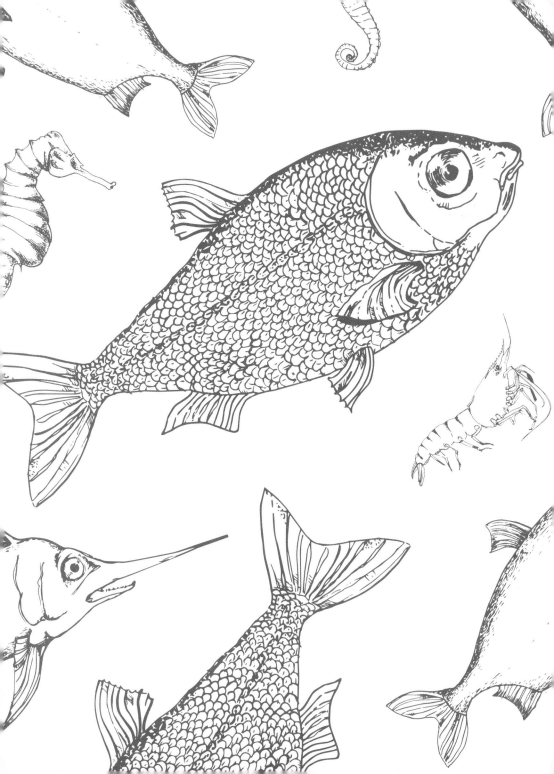

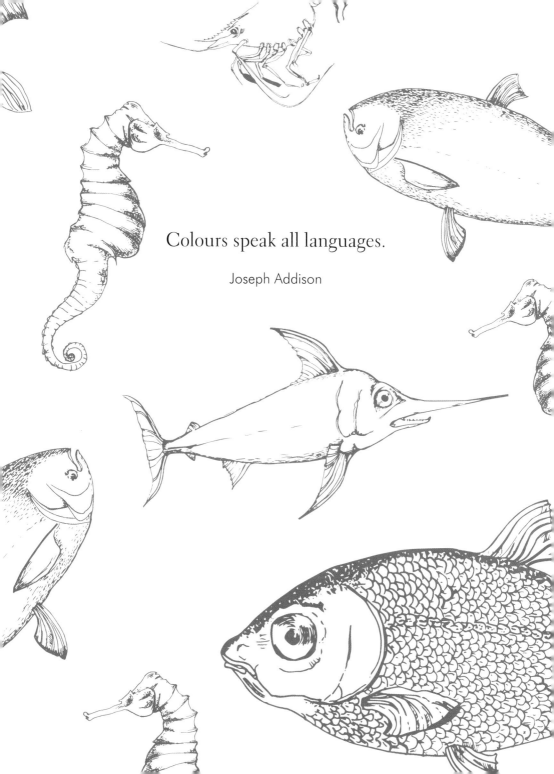

Colours speak all languages.

Joseph Addison

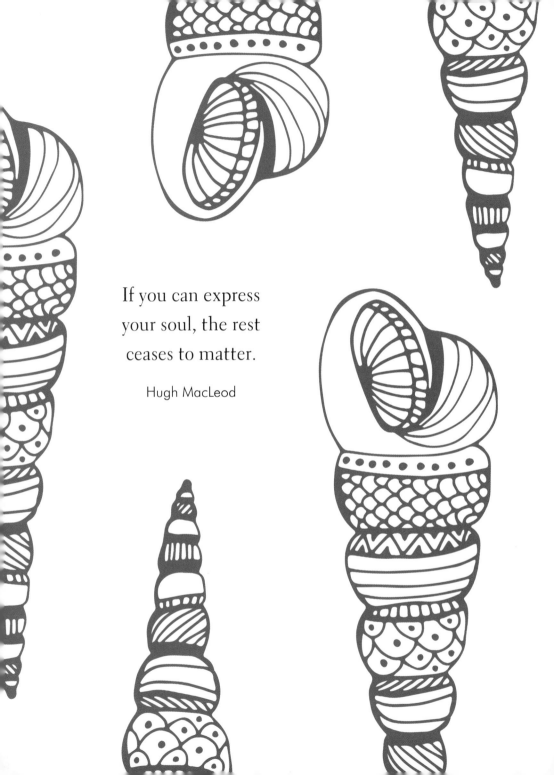

If you can express
your soul, the rest
ceases to matter.

Hugh MacLeod

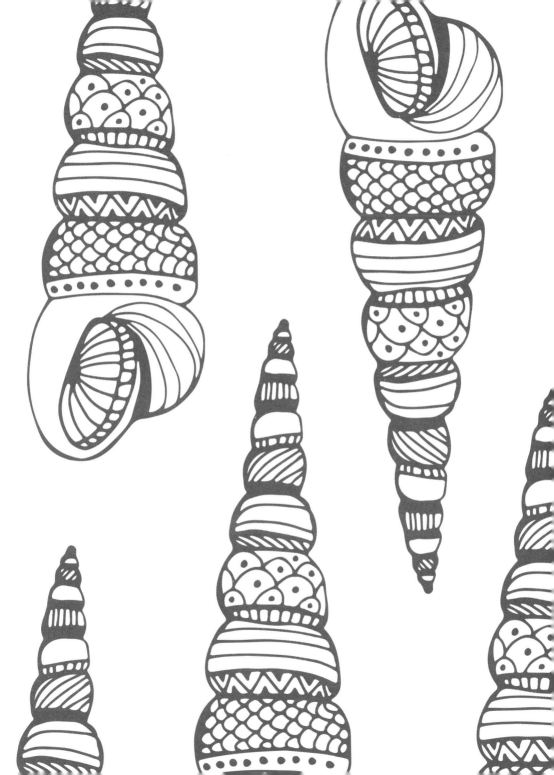

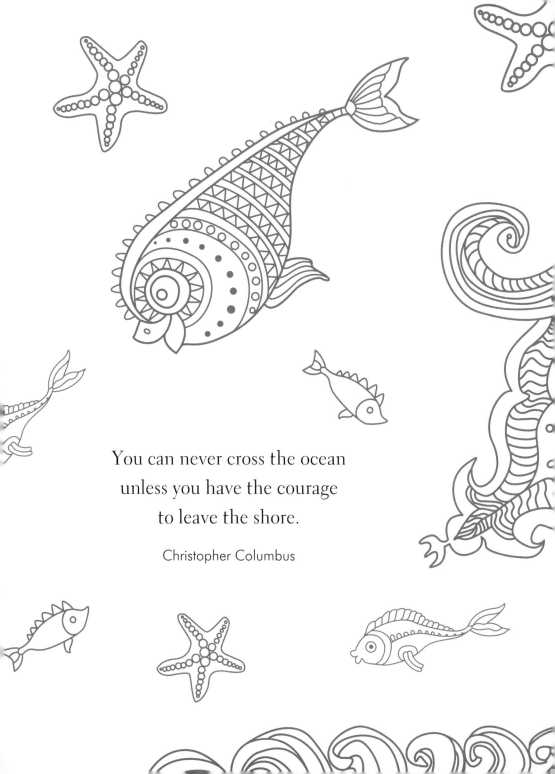

You can never cross the ocean
unless you have the courage
to leave the shore.

Christopher Columbus

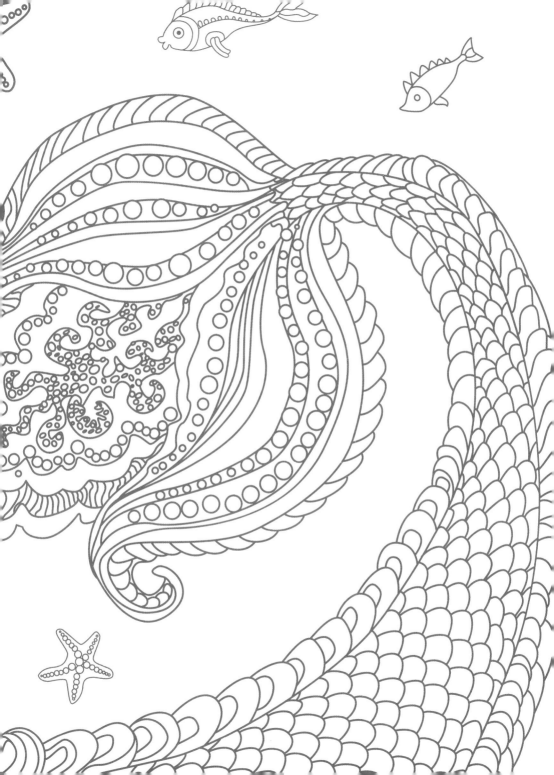

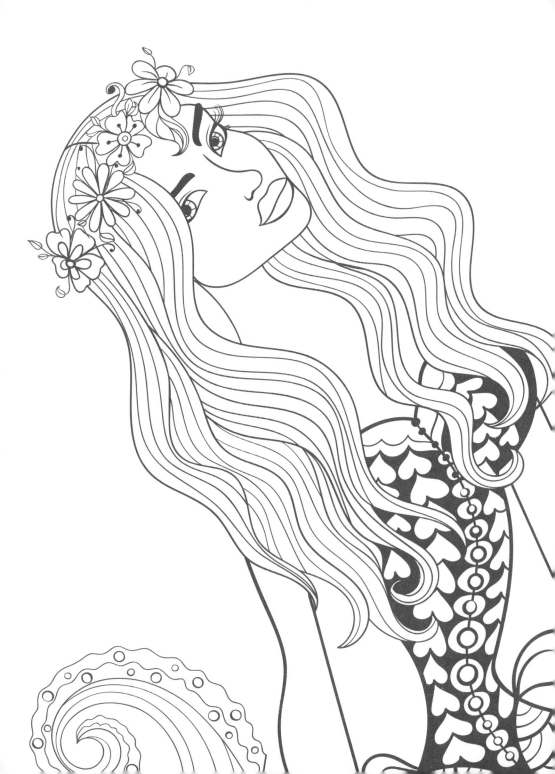

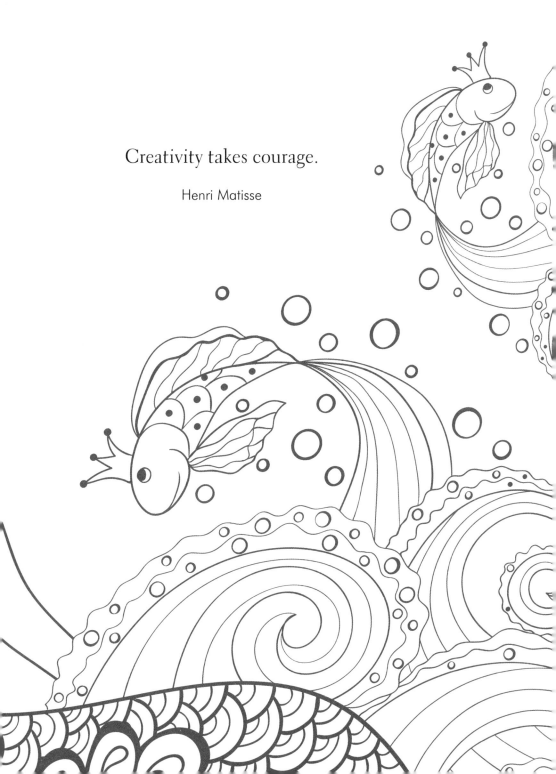

Creativity takes courage.

Henri Matisse

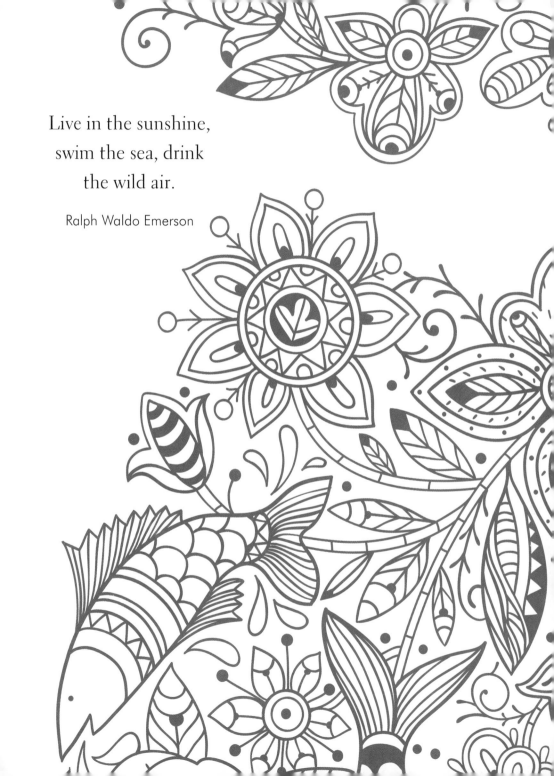

Live in the sunshine,
swim the sea, drink
the wild air.

Ralph Waldo Emerson

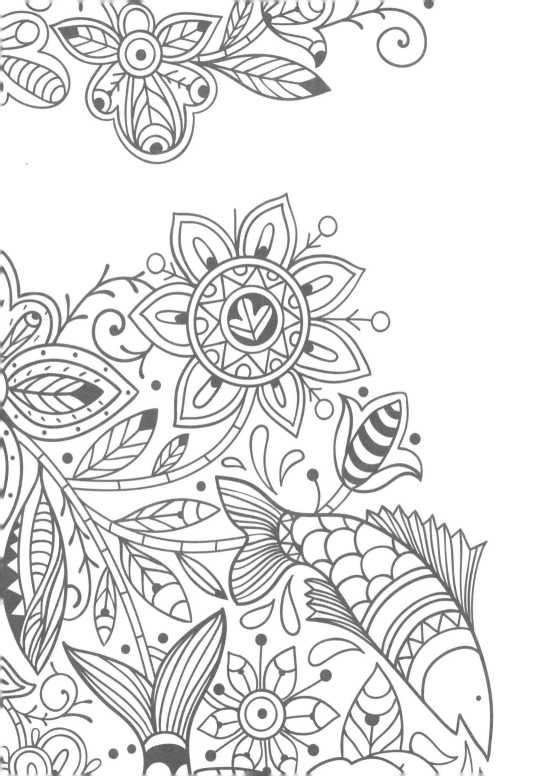

If you're interested in finding out
more about our products, find us on
Facebook at **Summersdale Publishers** and
follow us on Twitter at **@Summersdale**.

www.summersdale.com

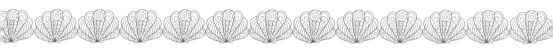

Summersdale Publishers Ltd
46 West Street
Chichester
West Sussex
PO19 1RP
UK

www.summersdale.com

Printed and bound in the UK by Bell & Bain Ltd, Glasgow

ISBN: 978-1-909865-26-6

Substantial discounts on bulk quantities of Summersdale books are available to corporations, professional associations and other organisations. For details contact general enquiries: telephone: +44 (0) 1243 771107 or email: enquiries@summersdale.com